BOOM

Boost Our Own Metabolism

BOOM! Back to Good Health

Harry A. Oken, MD, FACP

Stephen C. Schimpff, MD, MACP

"The future of American medicine will be centered around prevention and our ability to motivate patients to adhere to lifestyle changes, regular exercise programs, stress reduction techniques, and therapeutics that improve the duration and quality of life. In BOOM!, a comprehensive guide to improving your health, Dr. Oken and Dr. Schimpff share their tested philosophy on how to live a longer and better life. Members of the medical community — and our patients — are the lucky beneficiaries of their singular expertise and their combined decades of experience as practicing physicians. I commend Dr. Oken and Dr. Schimpff for sharing their unique and valuable perspectives, and for helping us all to live healthier and more rewarding lives."

Christopher O'Connor MD MACC
President and Executive Director, Inova Heart and Vascular Institute
Editor-in-Chief, Journal of the American College of Cardiology: Heart Failure

"In the exceptional book, "BOOM," Drs. Oken and Schimpff will take you on a sensational journey to improve your overall well-being. They use their expertise to simplify the complex science behind the four key pillars of health: nutrition, exercise, sleep, and stress. By giving you a clear understanding of the pillars, they will guide you through their straightforward program with diagrams, tips, and goals. I will be recommending this notable book to my patients, family, and colleagues!"

Robin West, M.D.
President, Inova Musculoskeletal Service Line
Lead Team Physician, Washington Nationals
Head Team Physician, Washington Redskins
Associate Professor, Georgetown University Medical Center & Virginia Commonwealth University School of Medicine

BOOM

Other books by Dr. Schimpff for a general audience:

The Future of Medicine: Megatrends in Health Care That Will Improve Your Quality of Life

Alignment: The Key to the Success of the University of Maryland Medical System

The Future of Health-Care Delivery: Why It Must Change and How It Will Affect You

Fixing the Primary Care Crisis: Reclaiming the Patient-Doctor Relationship and Returning Healthcare Decisions to You and Your Doctor

Fortune Seekers in the Promised Land: A Tale of Exploitation and Development in the Canaan Valley and Blackwater Region of West Virginia

Longevity Decoded: The 7 Keys to Healthy Aging

DEDICATION

For my wife and daughters —
Janet, Rachel, Stacey and Lindsey

For my wife, daughter and her family:
Carol, Becky, Brian, Ben and Bruno

The Action Step

This book is also dedicated to all of our patients and everyone who is interested in improving their life by addressing their health. We know that everyone — whether lean, overweight or obese — pauses periodically, maybe daily, weekly or monthly, and thinks, "What can I do to feel better, move better, sleep better, have a better outlook and live longer?" It is at those very moments that you are vulnerable enough to move forward with a change. It starts with an intention. The intention allows the contemplator to move into action. Action is the first step to building willpower, and willpower begets change — BOOM!

A Note on COVID-19

We wrote this book largely before the advent of the current coronavirus pandemic. We had in mind that most of you would spend one day per week at a gym for the HIIT exercise program and one day doing HIIT at home. But you can do both at home with a bit of creativity. All of the other advice on a quality diet, exercise, stress management and sleep are appropriate no matter where you are.

You may be spending time now sheltering in place, social distancing, following good hand hygiene practices and doing other steps to protect yourself and others. BOOM is the perfect antidote for long periods of isolation, and now is a great time to adjust your lifestyle and habits to become more ideal. You will feel better, be healthier and better deal with the stresses of COVID-19.

If you are finding it hard to maintain your resilience in face of the current pandemic, you might find this article by Dr. Schimpff helpful:

https://bit.ly/2xn9joE

Meanwhile, follow the BOOM plan and be pleased with your successful results!

CONTENTS

PREFACE

Welcome. By picking up this book, you have made the first step toward improving your health and enjoying a longer life with fewer serious diseases.

Going back just a century or less, our grandparents and great-grandparents had many fewer chronic diseases than what we develop today. These are the diseases that now cause most disabilities and deaths, such as heart failure, stroke, cancer, diabetes and Alzheimer's, along with high blood pressure and obesity. Modern medicine can do wonders in taming their effects but can rarely cure them. But you can prevent them and, if caught early, possibly even reverse them.

One hundred years ago, there were few packaged, prepared or processed foods and no fast food restaurants, but today they are the mainstays of our diet with high sugar, fat and salt content. Our ancestors ate two or three meals each day, prepared at home from fresh, local ingredients raised or grown in a manner today we would call organic. They rarely snacked. Today our foods are from long distances, not picked at the peak of ripeness, not organic and less often prepared at home. Meats are from penned, grain-fed animals, not ones that grazed in the fields and fish are not wild caught but farmed raised. Eggs come from hens kept in cages their entire lives, not from ones pecking and scratching in the soil. In addition to the typical meals eaten on the run, often in the car and not at a table with friends and family, we enjoy a mid-morning coffee with a pastry, an afternoon break with some cookies, and a late-night bedtime repast of ice cream. In other words, we eat about six meals per day.

Our forebearers were on the move all day long, not necessarily doing strenuous exercise but moving nonetheless. Today we drive to work, sit at a desk all day and drive back home where we sit to watch television.

Our ancestors went to bed when the sun set and arose with the sun. They slept soundly. Today's Americans are chronically short on sleep and even feel guilty about getting more than six hours per night.

Certainly, our grandparents had stresses in life, and many were persistent. But they accepted that life came with its adversities and managed them as best they could. Somehow, even with all that they had to do every day, they found time to sit back for a few minutes and contemplate life. Today everyone is chronically stressed, beginning in our teenage years and extending throughout life. We have more time-saving devices yet have less time to relax, contemplate and enjoy life.

Some of our forebearers smoked, but not many did. Smoking became popular once cigarettes could be machine-made and marketed to a wide audience. Soldiers during WWII were given free packs of cigarettes and the habit was formed. Smoking was considered not only socially acceptable but also manly — witness the Marlboro Man. Soon thereafter, it became acceptable for women to smoke as well, hence Virginia Slims' marketing tagline, "You've come a long way, baby." Fortunately, smoking has declined from its peak of about 45 percent of the population to about 17 percent today, but those who do smoke can anticipate a decade of life lost.

This book will explain the importance of what you eat and when you eat it, how and how much you move, how you sleep and how you manage chronic stress. Addressing these, which we call the "four pillars of health," and assuming that you do not smoke, will assure you of a lifetime of good health and wellness. It is imperative that you address all four together. Fixing just one will never be enough, otherwise you will shortly feel discouraged and the results will be unsatisfactory. To have true health, you need to maximize all four. You will feel better, have more energy and enjoy life to its fullest. It will be a journey of a lifetime of changed habits, replacing the old with the new. It will require your full attention and discipline. But it is not all that difficult, and the end results will be well worth the effort.

This book is based on a program developed by Dr. Oken in Columbia, Maryland, and presented at his local health club for the past six years. The program works. However, it does require diligence. Many who participate do so after some type of life event that convinces them it is now a necessity to change their lifestyle and take charge of their health. Sometimes it is an illness, a heart attack, the death of a loved one, or being told by a spouse that it is time to change — or else. There are also those who are overweight, sluggish, or do not feel like they did years ago and want to get a sense of health and wellness back again. The reason does not matter as long as the individual feels that he or she wants to make the change and is willing to engage fully. When that is the case, as it has been for about 60 percent of those who start the program, the results are excellent and enduring. However, we emphasize that the fear of dying or illness is not sustainable. It can be an initial instigator for action, but what we have found is that once involved, you will find greater energy, enthusiasm, stamina and reduced stress, making it is easy to maintain what you have achieved. You have no reason to revert because you feel better and want to continue with the "new you." As we progress in the chapters ahead, we will use examples of individuals who had high motivation and excellent results yet others who, for whatever reason, could not make the lifestyle changes needed to be successful.

You can read this book straight through in less than a few hours, and that might be a good idea so you get the overall concepts in mind quickly. Then return to the beginning and get started on the actual BOOM program. Each chapter builds on the last, and each concludes with a specific set of instructions for you to follow. Although the program is iterative, it starts with many of the basics, so be sure to follow along carefully and with diligence right from the beginning.

Remember as you think about starting BOOM that today the most common diseases and the ones that cause death are chronic conditions such as heart disease, diabetes, cancer, Alzheimer's and obesity. These illnesses, once they develop, are difficult to manage, expensive to treat and, in general, persist for life. What is important to realize is that they are mostly lifestyle-related. Yes, genetics plays a part but a relatively small part. Genes need not be your destiny. Following the precepts of BOOM will slow the aging process and largely prevent these chronic diseases. The result will be a longer, healthier life. That's something to strive for!

If you have not already worked to improve and maintain your health, now is the time. Put your health first, before everything else. Sound selfish? It is actually *selfless*. If you take care of yourself, you can take care of the people you care about: your spouse, your children, your friends and everyone else.

BOOM can and will change your life for the better. We are here to guide you. Perhaps the most important thing you can begin with is the recognition that you have the power to be successful and have a healthier future, one where wellness is the mark of success. Think of the power you have like a light switch. Flip it up to "on." You can do it just like that. BOOM!

FIRST THINGS FIRST

Before proceeding, it is important to recognize that we are offering healthcare information, not personal medical advice. We cannot be responsible in any way for adverse occurrences or circumstances. For actual personal health advice, you need to confer with your own primary healthcare provider. It is critical that you obtain explicit permission to participate. Your doctor, for example, might advise you not to engage in some of the exercises herein. Or you may be told to avoid certain dietary recommendations because of interactions with drugs that you are taking such as blood thinners or statins.

Once you have your doctor's go ahead and if you are still ready, then let us begin.

CHAPTER 1: INTRODUCTION AND AN OVERVIEW ON GETTING HEALTHIER

"If you do not change direction, you may end up where you are heading." - Lao Tzu

Jennifer had been a good-looking teen and young woman but now at age 45 had gained many extra pounds. One day while having lunch with her best friend Ellen at a neighborhood Italian restaurant, she was dipping her warm bread into the garlic-infused olive oil and thinking about her forthcoming chicken parmesan over pasta when Ellen looked her in the eye and said, "Jennifer, we have been friends for a long time and I don't want to hurt your feelings, but there is something I need to tell you. Something only a friend would do for a friend. Please don't be angry." Jennifer looked up and said that, of course, she would not be angry. Ellen then told her, "You are no longer the vivacious, energetic soul you had been, and frankly, look bad and have gotten fat." Jennifer was taken aback and hurt, but deep down, she knew it was true. These were harsh words that went to her core. "Ellen, I am hurt but you are right, and I know it, but I just don't know what to do. I have long realized I'm well overweight, and you know I have tried various diets with no real lasting success. I just don't know what to do." "Maybe," Ellen offered, "you could try that program at the local health club called 'BOOM.' I checked into it before lunch and found that they are having some good results — results that last. And they are now taking reservations for the next set of sessions starting in a few weeks."

Jennifer is not unusual. About two-thirds of Americans are overweight. Many Americans have high cholesterol, high blood pressure and high blood sugar. Diabetes is becoming an epidemic. And equally important, many people do not feel "up to snuff." Most would like to resolve these issues but tend to expect the doctor to offer a prescription or two. The notion that modifying your lifestyle could prevent or resolve these issues seems far-fetched and, even if possible, seems like too much effort in a life of too little time. The result is stasis with no action at all.

"If We Could Give Every Individual the Right Amount of Nourishment and Exercise — Not Too Much and Not Too Little — We Would Have Found the Safest Way to Health." - Hippocrates

This program, which we call BOOM (Boost Our Own Metabolism), uses scientific principles and medical evidence to attain and improve your overall health. If you follow our suggestions, you will see an increase in your lean body weight and a reduction in your fat weight. You will feel stronger, lighter and more energetic. You will definitely be healthier, and you will slow the aging process so you can live longer. At the same time, you will reduce the risk of many chronic illnesses, which are the diseases that cause most of today's disabilities and death.

Success depends on you. It takes personal discipline. And there is only one type of discipline, as General George Patton said: "Perfect Discipline." That said, the changes to your lifestyle that we recommend are not really difficult, and once you have made the switch, it will be relatively easy to maintain them. It does take persistence, and the initial change can be daunting since you (like almost everyone else) have developed certain adverse habits that are ingrained in your daily living.

Being healthy and maintaining wellness is an ongoing, never-ending project for all of us. It never stops. Being healthy is all about moderation and lifestyle and focusing on *The Big Four*, as listed below.

The Big Four boast many benefits, such as strengthening your immune system. Importantly, if your immune system is healthy, you are tipping the scale, so to speak, toward aging gracefully rather than decaying as you age. You will be more resistant to cancer, cardiovascular disease, diabetes, Alzheimer's disease and numerous other complex chronic illnesses.

Here are The Big Four:

- Sound nutrition

- Appropriate regular exercise

- Enhanced, healthy sleep

- Management of chronic emotional stress

Maintaining wellness and getting healthy is primarily based on what you eat, so we will focus a lot of time and attention on diet. It is the first among equals in our four pillars of health, and all four are absolutely essential.

Let us begin with a brief overview. We will return to all of these points as we proceed.

Food can be loosely divided into macronutrients (carbohydrates, fats and proteins) and micronutrients (vitamins, minerals and other critical chemicals needed for health). The three types of macronutrients contain energy that your cells use. Originally derived from the energy of the sun and converted by plants using chlorophyll into macronutrients, this energy is transferred to you by eating plants or eating animals that have eaten plants. Your gastrointestinal system breaks these macronutrients into their constituent parts: simple sugars from carbohydrates, fatty acids and glycerol from fats, and amino acids from proteins. These can be absorbed into the bloodstream and circulated to the cells of your body where they are used.

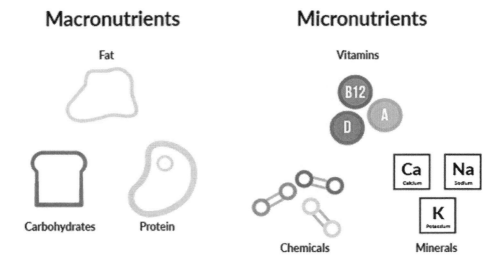

Macronutrients

Fat

Carbohydrates   Protein

Micronutrients

Vitamins

B12

D   A

Ca | Na
Calcium | Sodium

K
Potassium

Chemicals   Minerals

Micronutrients are substances or chemicals that your cells need to carry out their metabolic and physiologic functions. Usually, they are needed in only small or even trace quantities and hence are called micronutrients. Like the macronutrients, the micronutrients are found in the foods you eat. They include vitamins A, B1, B2, B3, B5, B6, B8, B9, B12, C, D, E, K and minerals such as calcium, magnesium, chlorine, phosphorus, potassium and sodium. Those needed in trace amounts are iron, copper, zinc, iodine, manganese, chromium, cobalt, and selenium and so-called phytochemicals such as carotenoids and flavonoids. Some would also include in this list the essential amino acids and essential fatty acids, which the body cannot create from the foods you eat, including the amino acids tryptophan, leucine and phenylalanine and the omega-3 and omega-6 fatty acids.

For the most part, you obtain immediate energy from carbohydrates in the foods you eat once they are broken down into simple sugars. One of these is glucose. It is the major source of energy that cells use and requires insulin to help it enter the cell. Energy enters the mitochondria (often referred to as the "power centers" of cells), where energy properties are transferred to a chemical called ATP and can be used by the cell for its various functions, such as muscle contraction or brain cell action. Most of these cellular reactions require the assistance of various micronutrients such as vitamins.

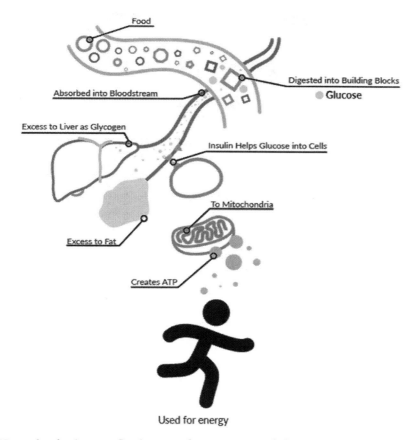

Food

Digested into Building Blocks
Glucose

Absorbed into Bloodstream

Excess to Liver as Glycogen

Insulin Helps Glucose into Cells

To Mitochondria

Excess to Fat

Creates ATP

Used for energy

Your body has a finely tuned system to deliver nutrients to cells. When you drink a soda, your brain instantly realizes that calories are on the way, and it sets a variety of responses in motion. First, the glucose (sugar) level in your bloodstream rises quickly. Next, a message goes to the pancreas to release insulin so the glucose can enter, for instance, a muscle cell that needs energy right then. Glucose in the bloodstream that is not needed at that moment is sent to the liver, where it is stored as a compound called glycogen. This keeps the level of glucose in the circulation at a fairly steady level of about 70 to 100 mg/ml. If those muscle cells need added glucose, insulin helps it move from the bloodstream to the cells and concurrently converts some of the glycogen back to circulating glucose, thereby keeping the blood sugar level nearly constant.

If you eat enough foods that convert to glucose and cause the excess to overflow the liver's glycogen storage capacity, the remaining glucose is stored in the liver as fat or in fat cells. These fat cells can be anywhere but are predominately in the abdominal (belly) area. Our ancestors relied on this stored fat to carry them over during periods when food was not readily available. Then, once their liver glycogen stores were depleted, the fat stored in the liver was converted back to glucose, as was the fat in the fat cells in the abdomen. That fat was also converted and released as small particles called ketones, which could also be used directly by cells as an energy source (more on that later).

Today, you probably never go hungry for any length of time, so the fat built up in the fat cells just stays there and continues to increase as you consume more calories than expended. As this little bit of fat becomes larger and larger, it produces a variety of chemicals that induce inflammation. This low-grade continual and persistent inflammation is harmful to many areas of the body, especially the coronary arteries of the heart and cells in the brain. Combined with other insults, the long-term results can be a heart attack or Alzheimer's disease.

This excess fat in the belly has recently come to be called "overfat." It is unhealthy and needs to be addressed.

One way to address it is through movement, yet Americans have become sedentary. Most of us no longer work in the fields or in the factory; we drive to work, sit at a desk, drive home and sit to watch television. The human body needs to move — lack of movement causes multiple adverse consequences, including an increased risk for heart disease, diabetes, stroke, high blood pressure, high cholesterol, Alzheimer's disease and some cancers. Movement uses energy and eliminates many of the harmful chemicals produced by the fat cells that cause inflammation. If you look at the so-called "Blue Zones," which are five areas of the world with a high proportion of centenarians, one of the consistent findings is near-constant movement from sunup to sundown. You need to do the same.

We all get scared if we see a big truck barreling down the road toward us. We run for the curb. We feel our heart race, breathe rapidly and have tightness in our muscles. Maybe you can sense the sudden adrenaline/epinephrine rush. It is an immediate response of your body to save your life. Once the threat has passed, you settle down. This is completely normal. However, low-grade stress is less noticeable, and when it is chronic from an unpleasant work setting, for instance, your body constantly releases low levels of acute stress chemicals such as epinephrine and cortisol. This is unhealthy, creates inflammation and predisposes you to a number of diseases such as heart disease and Alzheimer's. Unfortunately, many adults have such chronic stress most of the time. Bottom line, you need to get your stress under control. It is essential.

Sleep is also important for good health, but most people do not get enough. During sleep, your brain organizes the day's events as longer-term memories, prepares the brain to engage in new learning the next day, cleanses itself of toxins, works out problems that caused emotional turmoil during the day, and metabolizes excess adenosine, which left unabated, causes sleep pressure. Inadequate sleep adds to inflammation and works with your stress, lack of exercise and excess fat to damage critical areas of your body.

In the pages to follow, we will show you how to address each of these four pillars of health. With diligence, you can enjoy good health and live a long, pleasant life.

Jennifer decided to get involved and, as you will see as we chronicle her time with BOOM, did very well, both in the short-term and over the next few years. However, she certainly had her up and down days. You may as well, but the end result is well worth it.

CHAPTER 2: ADDRESSING OVERFAT

"Change the way you look at things, and the things you look at change." - Wayne Dyer

Jennifer made an appointment with her primary care physician. After being evaluated, she sat down in the doctor's office. He told her, "Your height is 5'7" and your waist is 36" or more than half of your height. Think back to geometry class in high school — the area of a circle goes up fast as the circumference goes up. And of course, that just refers to a single plane; we have to think more in terms of volume. Truth be told, you carry a lot of fat in your belly." He also told her that her blood pressure, cholesterol and HbA1c (hemoglobin A1c) levels were all elevated. "What's HbA1c?" she asked. "It's a measure of your average blood sugar levels over the past three months. Even though your fasting blood sugar was near normal, the HbA1c at 5.9 tells us that your blood sugars are often too high during the day. It may mean that you have some degree of insulin resistance, which is one of the first steps toward diabetes. I could give you prescriptions for each of these three issues, but instead, let's see what you can accomplish with the BOOM protocol. Lifestyle modifications should always be the first approach. My problem is that most patients won't give it a really good try. So, I am delighted you are committed. Go for it! And let's get together again in a few months to see how you are doing."

One-third of Americans are overweight, and another one-third are obese — that is two-thirds of us! Teenagers are now frequently overweight and often obese. Even young children are now growing up fat. It is a national epidemic of serious proportions and is only getting worse every year. Being overweight or obese is not just a cosmetic issue; fat produces many chemicals that damage your body on a slow but consistent basis, day after day, year after year. Eventually, it causes overt disease.

There is a new term coming into use — "overfat." Obviously, those who are overweight and obese are overfat. Even if you have a normal body mass index (BMI), your hip-to-waist ratio is within "normal limits" or the scale says you are still at your high school weight, you may still be overfat. It turns out that about two-thirds of those thought of as having an appropriate weight are still overfat. To learn more, read the article in this endnote.[1]

So, what is overfat and what happens if you are overfat? How can you tell if you are overfat? If two times your waist measurement is equal or greater than your height, you are overfat. The figure below shows this graphically. If you are a 5'10" man (70 inches) and your waist is 35 inches or more, then you are overfat. A 5'4" woman (64 inches) should have a waist size less than 32". And remember, these are *maximum* waist sizes, not ideal waist sizes!

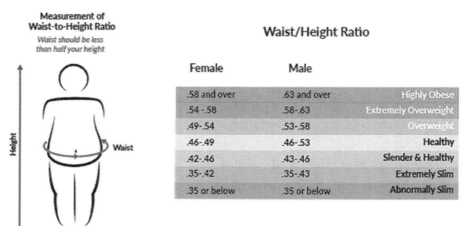

Measurement of Waist-to-Height Ratio
Waist should be less than half your height

Height

Waist

Waist/Height Ratio

Female	Male	
.58 and over	.63 and over	Highly Obese
.54 - .58	.58 - .63	Extremely Overweight
.49 - .54	.53 - .58	Overweight
.46 - .49	.46 - .53	Healthy
.42 - .46	.43 - .46	Slender & Healthy
.35 - .42	.35 - .43	Extremely Slim
.35 or below	.35 or below	Abnormally Slim

Essentially, overfat sets you up for an increased risk of a host of problems as shown below by this diagram:

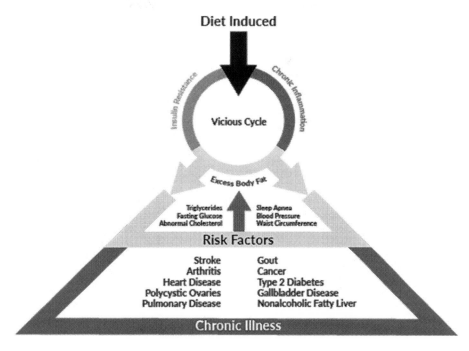

Diet, not only what you eat and how much you eat, but when you eat and how often you eat, is what leads to having too much fat in your body, especially an increase in your waist circumference. This excess fat leads to insulin resistance and chronic inflammation throughout various organs. The combination of insulin resistance and chronic inflammation, in turn, leads to metabolic syndrome, which is defined as any three of the following: high blood pressure, high cholesterol, high triglycerides, high blood sugar and excess belly fat. These factors predispose you to type 2 diabetes, heart disease, stroke, cancer and many other diseases.

When you eat any carbohydrate, it is reduced to sugar in the intestines and absorbed as glucose. If the body does not need more glucose right then, it is stored as glycogen, and if those stores are full, then it is stored as fat, mostly in the belly.

The core therapy for cholesterol management and many other issues such as elevated blood sugar and blood pressure, gout, sleep apnea and pain associated with osteoarthritis, is not a prescription for medication. The real therapy is attaining a weight that is healthy for you. Often, a small reduction in weight (just ten to fifteen pounds) will translate into a remarkable improvement in health and your sense of well-being. Even a reduction in weight of only one pound unloads four pounds per square inch on your weight-bearing joints, including the lower back.

Attaining and maintaining a healthy weight is a constant process of making adjustments. It is a challenging process. Perhaps the most significant obstacle is that your brain's pleasure center is continuously demanding that you seek calorie-dense foods that are almost always nutrient-lite. This mechanism evolved for prehistoric humans to avoid famine. Today, food is abundant and food technology has created unhealthy but alluring foods full of white flour, sugar, salt and bad fat — everything the pleasure center craves. The more we eat these easily stored *calorie dense* but *nutritionally limited* foods, the more we strengthen the pleasure center's hold on us. However, you can reset the pleasure center. Lifestyle changes in diet can modify the neurological networks and inhibit your cravings for unhealthy foods. This is the first step toward improving your metabolic health and your physiologic age. It takes hard work and discipline, but in days to weeks, you can tame the beast. But remember what General Patton said — it must be perfect discipline. Well, maybe not perfect, but darn close to it.

We like this quote from Michael Pollen in his book *The Omnivore's Dilemma*: "Eat food, not too much, mostly plants." By "food" he means real food, which is whole, fresh, local and not processed. And he adds "not too much." One need not be vegetarian, but the emphasis should be on plant-derived foods.

Here are a few tips for healthy eating. We will discuss each of these in more detail later, including how to calculate carbohydrates and protein.

- Eat a predominately plant-based diet. Try to get at least five servings of vegetables and appropriate serving sizes of fruit *every* day. On your plate, cover two-thirds with vegetables, with the last third or less reserved for proteins such as beans, fish or meat and some starches. Whenever possible, eat fresh, local vegetables picked at the peak of ripeness and preferably organic. This recommendation is certainly different from what many of us were brought up to expect and what we thought was healthy. We were told to eat meat or fish that covered about half of the plate and a starch like a baked potato, with the last quarter for some veggies. It is important to think in the opposite direction instead, with veggies first, probably two types per meal, no starch or at least not too much, and then a small portion of meat or fish.

- Eat in a low glycemic fashion, keeping daily carbohydrate intake to less than 50-60 grams per day (defined more below). This can be liberalized once the craving center of the brain calms down. You are probably eating more than 400 grams per day now, so this is a real cut and will be difficult for many people, but the result will be worth it.

- Minimize gluten-based white flour foods such as pasta, cereal, bread, pies, cakes, cookies, and yes, even pizza, as well as other complex starches such as rice and corn- and potato-based foods. These carbohydrate-heavy foods are converted during digestion straight to sugar.

- Eat fresh local fruits daily. Sure, fruit contains natural sugar, but the amount is fine unless you overdo it. Avoid excessive amounts of dried fruit. Although nutritious, we tend to eat more than we should. A small box of raisins is the equivalent of a whole bunch of grapes! You could eat four prunes but probably would never have four plums at one sitting.

- Avoid concentrated carbohydrates that are high in sugar, such as candy, cookies, cake, pudding, and ice cream. Fruit juices seem to be healthy, but they often have a high amount of sugar.

- Avoid soda, which is liquid candy. A typical twelve-ounce can of soda contains 39 grams of sugar (or slightly more than nine teaspoons!), which is more than a woman should consume in a full day and is essentially the maximum for a man. The American Heart Association recommends only 25 grams of sugar per day for women and 37 grams per day for men.

- Avoid sports drinks. They contain a high amount of sugar. So-called energy drinks are also high in sugar.

- Eat good fat. It is filling and, despite what we all read in the past, will not cause fat disposition in your body or elevated insulin levels. Examples of good fats include avocados, nuts, nut butters, olives and healthy oils such as olive oil. Fin fish like salmon, mackerel and sardines are loaded with healthy fats. Have some of these at least twice per week.

- Eat the correct amount of protein. Calculate this is as 0.5 grams of protein per pound per day of your ideal body lean weight. Good protein comes from beans and lentils, fish (preferably wild caught), poultry raised free-range, and meats from animals that are pastured and not penned and fed with corn and soybeans. We will help you calculate this later.

- Limit your eating times to two or three meals per day: breakfast, lunch and dinner. No snacking. Preferably, eat your largest meal midday rather than in the evening.

- Keep a food diary to track your daily intake. We all eat more than we think. Evidence-based scientific studies have shown that people who use a food diary are significantly more successful in their attempt to attain a healthy weight. You can keep a notebook with entries of everything you eat each day. It is recommended that you log every morsel of food placed between your lips, and it should take less than five minutes a day. Be complete and write "a third of a bag of chips" instead of "some potato chips." Not "a cookie" but "a large chocolate chip cookie followed by another." Do not be judgmental with yourself. The idea is to recognize and learn what you eat, not discipline yourself — at least not initially.

- There is a digital food diary that we recommend called MyFitnessPal, available at www.myfitnesspal.com and offered by Under Armour. It is free but has some built-in upgrades at a price; these can be helpful but are not necessary. MyFitnessPal can be used on your computer, tablet, or smartphone. (Please note that we have no affiliation with this company.) Once on the site, you will answer a number of questions about your demographics and activity. Additionally, you will select a realistic weight goal. MyFitnessPal will calculate the number of calories and carbohydrate grams you need each day.

In BOOM, the focus is on eating in a low glycemic manner, making you less of a carbohydrate-yearner and transition you to become an efficient fat-burner! We will write about this repetitively. For now, be aware of the carbohydrates that you are consuming. Our goal in BOOM is to keep total carbohydrate consumption to less than 50 grams per day for fourteen days. Remember that a can of soda contains 39 grams of sugar (a carbohydrate), so that single can is more than one-half of the total carbohydrates to be consumed each day. Doing this will likely be challenging at first as you reset the pleasure-craving center of the brain. After two weeks, you will transition to a higher level of carbs.

The exercise portion of this program is based on scientific evidence that says high-intensity interval training (HIIT) two times a week for less than thirty minutes per session will enhance your ability to burn fat at an efficient rate. The essence of HIIT is straightforward. Use an exercise bicycle or similar piece of equipment, warm-up for a few minutes, and then exercise as hard as you can for thirty seconds, followed by a ninety-second recovery period. Repeat this for eight cycles. After completing the eight cycles, take a few minutes at a modest pace as a cool down period, and then you are done for the day. At the start of this program, you will likely be unable to exercise aggressively for all eight of the thirty-second cycles, however, quite quickly you will find your endurance for high-intensity training will improve.

Here is what HIIT does. There are two types of muscle fibers — red and white. Aerobic training (like walking, biking, swimming or light jogging) recruits only the red muscle fibers, also called slow fibers. High-intensity training recruits the white muscle fibers, known as fast and ultrafast fibers. White muscle fibers have less blood flow and run out of energy quickly. The ensuing fatigue causes metabolic changes, including a spike in growth hormone, which will boost your metabolism — BOOM!

After working out, minimize your carbohydrate intake for at least two hours. Do not rehydrate with popular sugar-containing sports drinks, as this will counteract your goal of increasing your fat-burning metabolism, and it will also blunt the growth hormone levels that you just raised with HIIT. Rehydrate with water. It is also recommended you do HIIT exercise while fasting, unless you are a diabetic. It is okay to have water, coffee or tea prior to exercise, without sugar, of course. Do not drink juice, milk or a smoothie, as they are loaded with carbohydrates and will have a negative impact on what you are trying to accomplish.

Nutrition is crucial to seeing an improvement in your lean body weight as well. When combined with high-intensity exercise, you will become an efficient fat-burning machine. Over the course of this twelve-week program, you will learn the science behind high-intensity training as well as how to make proper nutritional selections that will boost your metabolism.

One more point. You should not feel ashamed or guilty if you are overweight. If 70 percent of Americans are overweight, then everyone is guilty. Perhaps the real culprits are those misguided individuals who have offered incorrect advice over the years. We will review the "wrong" and the "right" advice as we proceed.

Here is an observation from cardiologist Dean Ornish, based on his new book written with his wife, Ann. Ornish has shown that lifestyle adjustments can reverse heart disease and many other illnesses. "So, when people realize how much better they can feel when they make these changes to the degree they make them at any age, then it becomes self-reinforcing. Because these mechanisms are so dynamic, most people feel so much better so quickly, it really reframes the reason for making these changes from fear of dying or fear of something really bad happening, which is not sustainable, to joy and pleasure and love and feeling good, which really are." This is the promise of BOOM. You will feel better and have better health.[2]

BOOM! Here is your to-do list for the first week:

- See your healthcare provider and obtain clearance. Be sure to discuss the elements of HIIT or perhaps bring the pages above to show your doctor.

- Get started with your food diary. See Appendix 1 for a 10-day dietary recommendation

- Begin to reduce your carbohydrate intake and understand what 50-60 grams of carbohydrates encompasses.

- Begin a routine of thirty minutes of aerobic exercise six days per week. This can mean simply walking at a brisk pace.

Beginning next week, you will substitute HIIT for two of those days.

- If you do not have your own exercise bike at home, find a gym where you can do your HIIT program and where you can do twice-weekly resistance exercises with weights.

- Consider finding a few friends to join you on this journey. Participate and be infused with the group energy, which promotes self-discipline. Group support can be helpful, provided you each commit to not judging each other nor competing against one another. Otherwise, find a trusted friend, spouse or other relative to act as your buddy. This should be someone you trust who you can share your food diary with each week and talk about your efforts. This buddy needs to be supportive of your efforts, not judgmental.

Jennifer began her food diary. She was soon surprised about how many carbohydrates she ate each day. Most were foods that many would generally consider healthy — baked potato, pasta, cereal — but others included cookies, occasional soda and a morning pastry. Only 50-60 grams of carbohydrates was going to be a challenge. She began by cutting out sodas, ice cream, and snacks like cookies and pastries. That was difficult but not as hard as reducing pasta, sandwich bread and potatoes. And she would miss the Friday night pizza with friends.

CHAPTER 3: SUGAR, GROWTH HORMONE, INSULIN, AND YOUR HEALTH

"All things in moderation." - Ben Franklin

Jennifer began the BOOM program and found it difficult to do the exercise portion for more than three cycles. She had to slow down and not push so hard for the remaining five cycles. At first, she was discouraged that she could not do it, but the instructor reminded her that this is common. Most cannot do more than a few cycles at a high intensity at first. She was told it would get better each and every time.

Here is the short message of this chapter: Most carbohydrates are digested as glucose (or sugar), the most common energy source for your cells. When blood sugar rises after eating, insulin follows suit to help the glucose to enter cells. With too much glucose, the insulin pushes the excess into fat cells, especially in the belly. When you are intensely exercising after a prolonged overnight fast, your growth hormone rises. Growth hormone helps to build and maintain muscle fibers. But if you eat carbs too soon after exercise, the resulting rise in blood sugar and insulin negates the increase in growth hormone and its beneficial effects. Our message is that you should not eat after supper or before bed, and you should do high-intensity exercise while still fasting in the morning and avoid carbs for an additional two hours after that. What follows is a more detailed explanation.

When we eat food, it is digested into its basic components — proteins into amino acids, fats into fatty acids and glycerol and carbohydrates into simple sugars. These components, along with micronutrients such as vitamins and minerals, can be absorbed by the small intestines.

There are three simple sugars, also known as monosaccharides: glucose, fructose and galactose. Table sugar, or sucrose, is composed of one glucose and one fructose, making it a disaccharide. It is digested as its two component parts by the enzyme amylase.

Amylopectin is the carbohydrate in many starches like wheat flour. Amylopectin is composed of glucose molecules connected by the thousands. Digestion starts even before we take the first mouthful. Just the thought of food on the way begins to release saliva and is augmented by sight and smell. The saliva contains enzymes such as amylase, which begins the process of digesting the disaccharides and amylopectin.

Eating slowly and chewing are important to allow the early digestion process to be effective. The next stop is the stomach, which secretes acid that, along with the churning action, breaks down proteins, fats and carbohydrates into smaller and smaller pieces. Once that process is complete, the now-liquid substance, called chyme, is squirted bit by bit into the first part of the small intestine, the duodenum. Here new enzymes are released from the intestinal cells, pancreas and gallbladder. Combined, they continue the process of breaking down the chyme into the basic building blocks of amino acids, fatty acids and simple sugars like glucose and fructose. Glucose is the primary energy source for our cells found in our heart, muscles, brain and elsewhere.

With that as background, let us see how your exercise program will impact how you process the sugars. Recall from the previous chapter that in BOOM, we are targeting the super-fast white fiber muscles with our high-intensity interval exercise (HIIT). Training in an aerobic fashion like walking is healthy but only exercises our slow red muscle fibers. The white fibers need to be stimulated as well. Otherwise, they can decrease in number and atrophy. Short-burst HIIT exercise uses the red fibers but also recruits your white fibers and increases your growth hormone production. As you exercise, your body temperature increases, you sweat, your heart rate quickly elevates, and you feel your muscles burn … all in thirty seconds. By doing HIIT, you will see progress every week, and your ability to tolerate the exercise will increase.

Your job is to push yourself as hard as you can for the *entire* thirty seconds and find the resistance that makes this difficult. You may only be able to do this for the first couple of intervals, but as time goes on, you will make it the whole way.

This form of intense exercise, just for a few moments, not only impacts your muscles but also your growth hormone. From childhood to young adulthood, we regularly secrete growth hormone, particularly while we sleep. As we enter our 30s, our growth hormone secretion normally falls off. Most people in their late 20s and early 30s notice that they start to gain weight, particularly around their midsection. This is related to your diet, activity level and lower growth hormone levels, as well as higher basal insulin levels. When you enhance your growth hormone production, you increase your metabolism, and this helps you to mobilize fat and build muscle. This is one of the keys to the BOOM approach — drive up growth

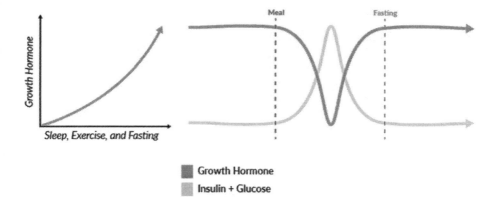

Sleep, Exercise, and Fasting

■ Growth Hormone
■ Insulin + Glucose

hormone and keep it there for a period of time so it can do its valuable work.

When we eat, digest and absorb sugars, glucose ("blood sugar") levels rise and insulin rises in response. Glucose is the basic energy for our muscles, brain and other organs, but it can only enter the cells with the help of insulin. However, the cells of muscles do not store glucose, for example, and they only take in what they need when they need it. The remaining glucose in the bloodstream above a basal level of about 100 mg/ml is stored in the liver as glycogen. Later, if the muscles need more glucose, it is taken from the bloodstream and enough of the glycogen in the liver is converted back to glucose to maintain that normal level. Think of it like a thermostat that keeps the house temperature steady, but here the system keeps the blood sugar level fairly constant so there is a steady supply of glucose for those muscle cells. If the liver's storage capacity for glycogen is completely at capacity from too much glucose after a meal or more likely a snack, glucose is then sent to fat cells where the glucose is converted and stored as fat — mostly around the midsection in the abdomen. This fat is okay in small quantities. This was how our ancestors long ago survived harsh winters when food was scarce. But too much fat sets up serious adverse consequences. Fat cells produce a variety of chemicals that are released into the bloodstream and travel to organs where they cause inflammation. Since these chemicals are constantly being released, day and night, the inflammation is perpetual and ultimately predisposes to disease, such as coronary artery disease, hypertension, diabetes, Alzheimer's disease and many others.

A diet loaded with carbohydrates that can be converted rapidly to glucose is called a high glycemic diet. High glycemic diets stimulate excess insulin production because of the rapidly increased blood glucose. There is a relationship between growth hormone and insulin secretion. With the rise in insulin, there is a drop in growth hormone. In other words, insulin levels and growth hormone levels are reciprocal to one another. Growth hormone levels can never be high when food intake is pushing up insulin. Growth hormone in adults is normally produced, albeit in small quantities, during the night if insulin levels are low. Exercise will rapidly increase output of growth hormone but, again, not if insulin is present. What this means to the BOOM program is that you want to go to bed with a low level of insulin and keep it low during your morning HIIT and beyond. Do this by not eating for about three hours before bedtime so the insulin has done its work and has returned to low levels, and then do not eat in the morning before the HIIT workout or for a few more hours after. Not eating foods that are high glycemic (and will raise the blood sugar levels and hence the blood insulin levels) is what you want to accomplish.

Bodybuilders have known this for quite some time, even if they did not understand the exact science. After a long muscle-exhausting, fatiguing workout, they consume high amounts of protein and no carbohydrates. By avoiding carbs and only having protein, they capitalize on the enhanced growth hormone secretion invoked by their heavy-duty muscle-fatiguing workout. They then build more muscle without storing fat. This is why you should not guzzle down a sugary sports drink after a high-intensity workout; it will shut off growth hormone and elevate your insulin level.

High glycemic beverages, like sports drinks, stimulate insulin secretion. High insulin levels promote fat storage, so when our insulin levels are high, we store fat. High glycemic foods include any food that is high in sucrose (table sugar) or fructose (fruit juice and all those foods that contain added "high fructose corn syrup"), as well as complex carbohydrates that may be gluten-based. Typical examples are juice, soda, candy, cookies, cakes and ice cream. Additional examples include "the whites" like pasta, bread, wheat-containing cereal, potatoes, and rice, because each is digested quickly into glucose, which is rapidly absorbed with resultant insulin secretion. Remember that when we do not need more glucose in our brain or muscles or elsewhere, but we have eaten foods that raise the glucose level in the blood, our insulin level will go up. This is the time when we store that extra glucose as fat. A healthy low glycemic diet consists of vegetables, fruits, good quality proteins and healthy fats with little sugar and only modest flour-based food. This limits the sudden sharp rise in blood sugar and promotes low insulin levels.

To recapitulate, we can enhance our metabolism by exercising in a fasting state and not having any significant amount of carbohydrates within two hours after high-intensity exercise. Use your best efforts to not eat anything after 7-8 p.m. On the morning of high-intensity exercise, be well hydrated with water, tea or coffee with no added sugar. If needed, have a small protein snack after your sessions. Try to not exceed 15 grams of carbohydrates within two hours of your high-intensity exercise. This will keep your insulin levels low and maximize the effect of growth hormone secretion invoked by white muscle fiber fatigue.

We will return to considering stress and sleep later, but for now, remember that reduced stress and restorative sleep also help to maintain and rehabilitate your immune system and control chronic stress. During the day, try to minimize your sitting. Get up every hour and walk around, or do some stretching, lunges or squats. Work standing up if you can. In addition to the aerobic cardiovascular exercise six times per week, add stretching and weight training two times per week. Again, more detail to follow.

BOOM! Week 2 Program

- Continue with the food diary.

- Reduce total carbohydrate to 50-60 grams per day; see Appendix 1. This likely will be hard at first, but over time you will be able to do it successfully. MyFitnessPal will help you with the calculations.

- Eat quality food, especially plenty of various fresh, local, simply-prepared vegetables, fruits, beans and lentils, good quality proteins and healthy fats as found in nuts and seeds, avocados, wild caught fin fish and olive oil.

- Reduce your consumption of added sugar to essentially zero. Avoid packaged and processed foods and fast food restaurants. Read labels. You will be surprised at how many foods have added sugars. Foods you thought were healthy, like yogurt, are inherently healthy, but many, if not most of those on store shelves, have added sugars along with vanilla or fruit that is supposed to attract you to buy.

- Continue your daily walks and twice-weekly resistance exercises.

- Begin the HIIT exercises twice per week at the gym using a stationary bike, treadmill, elliptical or rowing machine. Of course, at any time you are light-headed or dizzy – STOP! See Appendix 2.

If you want to do your second weekly HIIT workout at home instead of at a gym, you can consider this eight-minute alternative. It is *not* an alternative for at least once weekly regular HIIT exercise and, if possible, we strongly recommend that you do both at the gym.

- 20 seconds of jumping jacks

- 10 seconds rest

- 20 seconds run in place with high knees or jump rope without a rope

- 10 seconds rest

- 20 seconds of push-ups

- 10 seconds rest

- 20 seconds of mountain climbers*

- 10 seconds rest

- Repeat each step once more

* For the mountain climbers exercise, start in a plank position with arms and legs long for proper form. Keep your abs pulled in and your body straight. Squeeze your glutes and drop your shoulders away from your ears.

- Pull your right knee into your chest. As the knee draws to the chest, pull your abs in even tighter to be sure your body does not sag or come out of its plank position.

- Then switch and pull the left knee in.

- Continue to switch knees. Pull the knees in right, left, right, left — always switching quickly so you are using a "running" motion. As you begin to move more quickly, be in constant awareness of your body position to keep a straight line in your spine. Try not to drop your head and look forward.

CHAPTER 4: THE GLYCEMIC INDEX

"If God hadn't meant for us to eat sugar, he wouldn't have invented dentists." - Ralph Nader

"Yikes! My wife, Janet, makes the best carrot cake ever! I will have some today, but after that, it goes in the freezer for another time and day. Why? Because sweet, moist cake and cream cheese frosting signal the pleasure center in my brain to go wild for a couple of minutes as I eat, and a little after, I keep yearning for more. There is an explosion of neurotransmitters. And the more I have, the more I want."

"But ... I am in control of me, and you are in control of you. I know I will feel better in the long run by not eating concentrated carbs. And when I do decide to eat high glycemic carbs, those tasty but useless calories cause my blood sugar and insulin levels to rise and encourage fat storage rather than burning.

"And so, when I decide to eat those high glycemic carbs like my wife's carrot cake, I know I will need to work hard to burn some extra calories to pay it back! It might be a long walk, a hard workout in the gym, a swim, or just thirty squats by my desk throughout the day. You have to earn those treats."

Another strategy if and when you decide to have a high glycemic food like dessert is to control your portion size. It is not the initial bite that will do you in — it's the urge to finish the portion and maybe have a second. Also remember, if you have one or two bites and then distract yourself, 15 minutes later your brain will know the difference between having one bite instead of the whole thing.

So, our advice is to stop being a carb yearner and instead begin being a fat burner! Recognize those patterns and the effect of your brain's pleasure center and take control. We will write more about taking control in a subsequent chapter, but for now, let's learn more about high and low glycemic foods.

The Glycemic Index

The glycemic index provides a measure of the degree by which blood sugar levels rise after eating a particular type of food. High glycemic foods are the ones that are digested rapidly into glucose, which is then rapidly absorbed by the intestines into the bloodstream and causes insulin to spike. Low glycemic carbohydrates and other foods may also be digested into glucose but do so more slowly, largely because they are loaded with fiber. With these foods, insulin does not spike up and instead rises more slowly. Pure glucose has the highest glycemic index of 100 while olive oil is zero. A food with a high glycemic index will require higher levels of insulin as a response. Remember, high insulin levels promote the storage of calories as fat. Try to consume foods that have a lower glycemic index, which means plant food (non-starchy vegetables and fruits) and sources of healthy protein such as beans, lean meat, fish, seafood and poultry. And remember that fats are low glycemic as well, so do not be afraid to eat healthy fats such as avocados, nuts, seeds and olive oil.

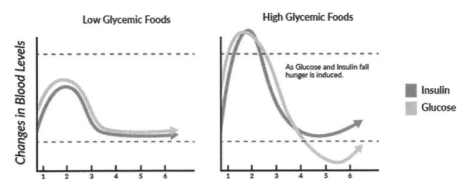

28

Gluten and Amylopectin

Gluten is a protein found in wheat. Gluten is co-joined in wheat (along with some other related grains such as rye and barley) with a complex carbohydrate-starch called amylopectin. Gluten is poorly digested by many individuals, but the amylopectin starch is rapidly digested in our bodies, first into glucose by amylase in the saliva and then with more amylase in the first part of the small intestine. The glucose is absorbed quickly into the bloodstream. This explains why two slices of whole wheat bread or one bagel have a very high glycemic index. It is counterintuitive, but those two slices of bread have 25 grams of carbs that produce glucose when digested. This is the same amount of carbs as a regular-sized Snickers bar, which has 27 grams!

Insulin Resistance

Eating a lot of sugar (such as candy or soda) or white flour-based food leads to high blood sugar, which in turn causes insulin levels to rise steeply. When this happens over and over again, it leads to diminished cell responsiveness to insulin. This is known as insulin resistance and is the beginning point of pre-diabetes and metabolic syndrome. It also leads to the creation of visceral belly fat, which in turn worsens insulin resistance. Fat can also accumulate in the liver and create a "fatty liver." This can inflame the liver and cause a condition called nonalcoholic fatty liver disease (NAFLD). As the country's epidemic of obesity has risen, NAFLD has become one of the major causes of cirrhosis (liver scarring) that leads to liver failure and even liver transplant.

Chronically spiking high blood sugar also damages the pancreatic beta cells that produce insulin. Over time, the pancreatic beta cells die and do not regenerate. Foods that increase blood sugar the most are the ones that cause the most toxicity. Remember that it is not just sugar of various types but the wheat-based foods that dominate our modern diet.

Carbohydrates are composed of starch, which has two components — amylose and amylopectin. Both are composed of glucose molecules linked together but in different patterns. Amylose takes time to digest whereas amylopectin digests readily. Rapid digestion means rapid blood sugar spikes followed by rapid insulin rises, and slower digestion means slower blood sugar and insulin elevations. High glycemic foods are those with high concentrations of amylopectin whereas low glycemic foods are the opposite.

Refining food, such as converting whole wheat to white flour, rolled oats, and other steps to produce processed foods like cereals, disrupts the natural amylose-amylopectin structures and leads to a higher glycemic index. On the other hand, fats and acids slow digestion of amylopectin. For example, an avocado with healthy fat content has a low glycemic index. A lemon with acid will also lower the glycemic index. Long slow cooking of a starchy vegetable means faster digestion. When a fruit ripens, it may have an increase in its glycemic index. For example, an unripe banana has a glycemic index (GI) of about 30 whereas a fully ripe one has a GI of about 50, still relatively low but certainly higher.

Here is a partial list of high versus low glycemic carbohydrates:

HIGH GLYCEMIC	LOW GLYCEMIC
Sugar in any form (table sugar or sucrose, fructose, honey, maple syrup, etc.)	Most fruits, in moderation
Watermelon, pineapple, overripe bananas, most dried fruits such as dates, raisins, prunes, apricots	
White flour-based foods – bread, pasta, pizza, cakes, pies, cookies, pastries, gravies, many breakfast cereals, instant oatmeal	Oatmeal (not instant), barley
Processed foods – These are usually	Nuts, olives, olive oil

based on refined flour, which has fiber and other nutrients stripped away.	
Boiled white potatoes, white rice, French fries	Sweet potatoes
Starchy vegetables such as canned or frozen corn, parsnips, winter squash	Non-starchy vegetables such as asparagus, artichoke, avocado, broccoli, cabbage, cauliflower, celery, cucumber, eggplant, greens, lettuce, mushrooms, peppers, tomatoes, okra, onions, spinach, summer squash, zucchini, turnips

Foods that are mostly fats or protein with minimal carbohydrates are generally low glycemic. Meat, fish, poultry and eggs are all low glycemic. So, too, are dairy products. Even though milk contains the milk sugar lactose, it also contains a high concentration of fats, which slows digestion and absorption of sugar.

To complicate matters some, the amount of any food eaten obviously has an impact on how much your blood sugar rises quickly. This has led to another term called glycemic load (GL). For our purposes, it is simply best to eat carbohydrates that have a low glycemic index and keep the total carbohydrates to less than 50 grams per day.

Recently, there has been great interest in reducing gluten-containing foods on the theory that this is a healthy approach to eating. It is but it is also important to realize why. Gluten is the protein in wheat but refined white wheat flour that has been stripped of its fiber and vitamins also contains lots of amylopectin that digests rapidly and is high glycemic. So, sticking to a diet of fewer high glycemic foods means avoiding white flour-based processed foods such as most cereals, breads, pastas, pizza, and obviously cookies, pastries, cakes and pies.

Do not become confused with gluten intolerance versus celiac disease. Celiac disease is an autoimmune disorder that begins in the small intestine and occurs in genetically predisposed people of all ages. It affects about 1 percent of Americans. Celiac disease can cause abdominal pain, discomfort in the digestive tract, increased intestinal permeability ("leaky gut") and altered bowel function. It can also have many systemic effects such as anemia, "brain fog," rashes, arthritis and other maladies. There is also a fairly common but unrelated condition that affects perhaps 10 percent or so of Americans known as gluten intolerance, which can also cause belly discomfort, bloating, constipation, diarrhea and reflux. Those with celiac disease must totally eliminate gluten from their diet. Those with intolerance generally find they feel better by eliminating or reducing gluten.

Lowering our intake of high glycemic foods, especially gluten-containing foods, can be very helpful in attaining a healthier weight and decreasing the likelihood of developing diabetes and cardiovascular disease. But remember, your key reason for replacing gluten-containing foods, at least for our purposes with BOOM, is to eliminate as many unnecessary high glycemic carbohydrates as possible. You do not want to replace gluten-containing foods with gluten substitutes such as rice starch or potato flour, as that is merely substituting one carb for another. Today there are many foods in the store labeled "gluten free," but the gluten has been replaced by something else and usually is another carbohydrate, including sugar. Gluten free is definitely not equivalent to "healthy." Read the labels carefully. Remember that eating a lower-carbohydrate meal will mean a smaller increase in blood sugar and a lower likelihood of developing insulin resistance.

When confronted with a situation in which you know you should not eat something, such as a plate of cookies brought to work by a coworker, learn to say out loud, "Thank you for offering, but I am not going to eat that cookie (or whatever)." The act of saying it adds weight to your decision. If it is said where others can hear you, it adds even more strength to your resolve, and they will respect you. You need not feel guilty that you are insulting your friend or coworker by refusing. It is your body, and your legitimate needs should take priority. Letting everyone know what your needs are and doing it verbally will engender goodwill and probably a bit of awe.

Remember, one of our key messages with BOOM is to reduce your total carbs. These are food products that can be used as energy, but once no more glucose is needed, the remainder is converted and stored as fat, mostly around your belly. And when food is high glycemic, it leads to rapid increases in insulin, which ultimately creates insulin resistance and diabetes.

BOOM! Week 3 Program

- Continue with the food diary. By using the MyFitnessPal app, you will likely discover that you are eating many more carbs per day than you imagined.

- Continue with total carbohydrates of 50-60 grams per day.

- Eat quality food, especially plenty of various fresh, local, simply prepared vegetables, as well as fruits, beans, lentils, good-quality proteins and healthy fats such as nuts, seeds, avocados, wild caught fin fish and olive oil.

- Reduce your consumption of added sugar to essentially zero. Avoid packaged and processed foods. Read labels — you will be surprised at how many foods have added sugars such as many yogurts.

- Stay away from fast food restaurants.

- Do not just think it, say it out loud so not only you but others will hear you: "I am not going to eat that donut!" It is very powerful.

- Continue your daily walks and two weekly resistance exercises.

- Move! Get up from your desk every hour, do some squats and get 7,500 to 10,000 steps every day.

- Continue the HIIT exercises twice per week at the gym using a stationary bike, treadmill, elliptical or rowing machine.

- Since you will not be doing your HIIT as part of an instructed class, consider the Tabata Pro app to help you with this challenge.

- Remember to go to the gym in a fasting state without breakfast and avoid eating for about two hours after your HIIT workout.

- Of course, at any time you are light-headed or dizzy — STOP!

CHAPTER 5: BURN, BABY, BURN WITH PROLONGED OVERNIGHT FASTING

"A little starvation can really do more for the average sick man than the best medicines and best doctors." - Mark Twain

Jennifer stuck with the program, pushing to get down to 50-60 grams of carbs per day though she found it difficult. But she was getting better at HIIT and could now do four of the eight cycles without letting up. She had always eaten a breakfast of cereal, milk and some fruit, plus coffee with milk and sugar for breakfast. Now she faced a new challenge — go to the gym without breakfast. She could still have coffee, but it had to be without sugar. Not only that, but the instructions were to avoid any food for about two hours after she finished her HIIT.

You can burn away that fat and feel much better. So far, you have learned about lowering your carbohydrate intake and you have begun the HIIT program. Now we will add in one more technique to help you burn off that fat — time-restricted eating, also known as prolonged overnight fasting. There is compelling information that overnight fasting/time-restricted eating can allow you to tap into your fat stores and become more efficient in metabolizing fat.

There is actually more to this. Even if you are not overfat and do not need to lose weight, intermittent fasting can be another key step in your approach to attaining better health. Along with fewer carbohydrates and HIIT, intermittent fasting may help you to reverse metabolic syndrome, type 2 diabetes, high blood pressure and high cholesterol and also prevent diseases such as Alzheimer's and Parkinson's. If that is not enough, you will feel better and have more energy!

Go back a few generations to when most Americans lived on the farm. They ate much differently than we do today. They did not have all the processed, packaged foods available now nor the fast food restaurants. They ate foods that were local, ripe and in season. Sweets were a treat; the sugar consumption then was minuscule compared to today's approximately 75-155 pounds (!) per person per year. Their major meal was usually at midday, and supper was a more limited affair. Most got up early and went out to milk the cows, collect the eggs and get started with farm work in general. The farmer came back in for a breakfast, which was comprised not of cereal but of eggs and some meat and perhaps a piece of whole grain toast with butter and a bit of jelly. Cream went into the coffee. All organic. Notice that, unlike today, the meal was taken later in the morning and was lower in carbohydrates but higher in healthy fats and protein. They almost never snacked as we do today. No morning donut, no midafternoon pastry and no late-night trip to the refrigerator. They ate two or, at most, three meals per day and did not feel the drive to eat additionally. Fasting was not thought of as such since it was just part of everyday life. Breakfast eaten later in the morning was just that — breaking the overnight fast.

Who told us that breakfast is the most important meal? The answer is Kellogg's!

Kellogg's began an advertising campaign back in the 1960s to convince Americans that they must have breakfast. And of course, the "breakfast of champions" was exactly what we did not need first thing in the morning — complex carbohydrates made largely with refined white flour. Although it may take longer for these carbs to convert to glucose than pure table sugar, convert they do with rising insulin levels and reduced growth hormone levels. Since you are not doing much other than sitting around the table eating, the excess glucose goes to the liver to replenish the glycogen that was used during the night.

Prolonged Overnight Fasting/Time-Restricted Eating

What is prolonged overnight fasting? Basically, it is not eating for about three hours between the evening meal and bedtime and then continuing to not eat until at least twelve hours after dinner or preferably a total of fifteen to sixteen hours. Remember that the term we use every day is "breakfast." It is literally breaking the fast from the night before. It is important to give some thought and follow-up to the concept that we should not eat for those twelve to sixteen hours. Here is why: The major point of time-restricted eating or fasting is to keep insulin levels low. It is during that time that body repair mechanisms can occur and fat, instead of glucose, can be used for energy.

The reason for not snacking after dinner and before bed with some ice cream is to assure that your insulin levels have returned to normal and stay down overnight. You do not want to go to sleep while insulin is still elevated. Some nuts and seeds would not elevate insulin levels, but avoiding any snack is best.

It takes at least eight to twelve hours to burn off the glycogen stores accumulated in your liver after eating throughout the day. This can occur once insulin levels are down. When they are up, the insulin is busy building up more liver storage of glycogen. Once the glycogen is used up, you can begin to use the fat stored in the belly for energy. But as soon as you begin to eat carbohydrates again, insulin increases and the liver rapidly begins the process of storing up glycogen. The use of fat for energy is dramatically curtailed. From your body's perspective, it is not necessary to use those fats for energy if carbohydrates are available. Glucose, if it is available, is always the default energy source for your cells.

Prolonged overnight fasting/time-restricted eating was not only common but the standard way of living in days gone by when snacks and sodas were not prevalent and people ate just two or three meals each day. They went to bed with the sun and got up with the sun. It was not called "fasting," but it was the norm. Today, prolonged overnight fasting/time-restricted eating means a dramatic lifestyle change for many, if not most people.

With time-restricted eating, the window of consumption of healthy food occurs within a nine-hour window, say, between 10 a.m. and 7 p.m. so you are fasting after 7 p.m. until 10 a.m. the next morning. Very quickly, most people will likely see a decline in their sugar cravings. Fasting helps to normalize insulin secretion as well as leptin and ghrelin levels (more on these later). Fasting also lowers triglycerides and, importantly, is associated with a reduction in chronic inflammation.

Fasting to keep insulin levels low, along with high-intensity exercise, improves your ability to burn fat. Doing high-intensity exercise in a fasting state while you are glycogen-depleted allows for an increase in growth hormone to boost your metabolism, build muscle and improve your fat burning.

Recall that growth hormone (GH) promotes muscle growth and boosts fat loss by increasing metabolism. It is well accepted that HIIT causes myokine release from skeletal muscles, which triggers a sustained release of GH.

Fasting also increases catecholamines, like adrenaline, which increases resting energy expenditure. Meanwhile, since you are not eating concentrated carbs first thing in the day, your insulin levels will not increase, and that allows stored fat to be burned for fuel.

Fasting also seems to improve cognitive function. Fasting in a glycogen-depleted state causes your fat cells to produce fatty acids and ketones, which are burned in the brain mitochondria in an efficient manner. Fasting increases brain-derived neurotrophic factor

(BDNF) as well. This protein activates brain stem cells and may protect you from Alzheimer's disease and Parkinson's disease.

One of the mechanisms that makes overnight fasting so effective for weight loss is that it provokes the natural secretion of human growth hormone, just like high-intensity interval training. The two together make for a powerful synergistic combination.

Take two groups of people in a controlled setting and give them the same total number of calories, with one group eating three meals and three snacks during a typical day and the other group limited to the same calories over three meals and ten hours. The calorie level is set so that the first group would gain some weight over the trial period. The first group gains weight as anticipated, but the latter does not. They eat the same total calories, but in the time-restricted eating group, the impact is much different. What this tells us, in part, is to follow our circadian rhythm. Eat during the day and keep it to two or three meals.

The circadian rhythm is not just about when you sleep and when you are awake and alert. All of your body's cells have their own circadian rhythm. They need a period of rest to do cell maintenance and repair and a different time for cell growth and development. The two do not occur together. Providing your cells with time for repair is a significant step to good health.

It is during that overnight "fast" that the body repairs itself by cleaning out the intracellular debris. Some research suggests that using the time-restricted eating pattern leads to lowered cholesterol, lowered blood pressure, lowered blood sugar and, if needed, lower weight or "overfat." These same studies suggest that the dose of blood pressure medications, diabetes medications and statins will all come down or even be eliminated over a period of months to a year with this approach. If these studies are borne out with further research, then this is the natural way to, at no cost, reduce or eliminate some of the most serious, disabling and expensive problems that beset Americans today — the very problems that lead to the diseases that cause death.

In a review of the literature on fasting by Patterson and Sears, they say: "Several lines of evidence also support the hypothesis that eating patterns that reduce or eliminate nighttime eating and prolong nightly fasting intervals may result in sustained improvements in human health. Intermittent fasting regimens are hypothesized to influence metabolic regulation via effects on (*a*) circadian biology, (*b*) the gut microbiome, and (*c*) modifiable lifestyle behaviors, such as sleep."[3]

In a study called "early time-restricted feeding," the subjects were given the same meals but taken either between 7 a.m. and 3 p.m. or between 7 a.m. and 7 p.m. The number of calories eaten was controlled and set to be about what each person needed for energy each day. On average, participants in neither group gained nor lost weight. But those who ate in the shorter eight-hour period each day soon had lower insulin levels, improved sensitivity to insulin and lower blood pressure. This approach of a longer overnight fast with the same food intake improved their metabolism. Fasting or time-

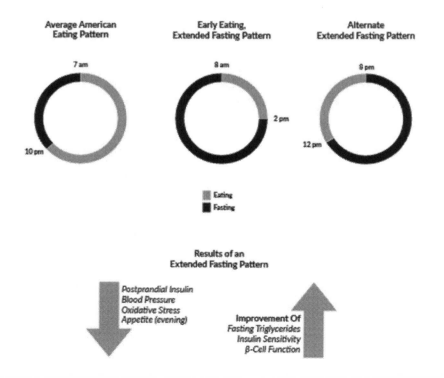

restricted eating improved health even though weight was not reduced in the study group.[4]

Contrary to what you were probably taught over the years, you do need to eat fats, but they need to be healthy fats. To repeat from earlier chapters, a few examples are nuts and seeds, nut butters, eggs, olives and olive oil, coconut oil, and avocados and avocado oil. Of course, cold-water fin fish like salmon, mackerel and sardines are loaded with healthy omega-3 fats. Animal meats raised entirely grass-fed in the pasture have omega-3 fatty acids as well but much less than fish. Dairy products from grass-fed cows have a healthier balance of unsaturated omega-6 to omega-3 fatty acids. Butter is mostly fat with about 400 different fatty acids, two-thirds saturated and one-third unsaturated.

Autophagy

What else happens when you fast? Autophagy, or the process cells use to eliminate cellular "leftovers," picks up. "Phagy" refers to eating and "auto" means self, so "autophagy" is the cell eating itself in a deliberate, needed manner. Think of it as a natural process that is highly regulated to take apart those elements in the cell that are no longer needed or are somehow "broken." Pictorially, imagine a "Pac-Man" engulfing unneeded materials — pieces of proteins, enzymes, mitochondria and other stray materials — which are then digested back into elemental compounds that can then be reused.

Fasting and sleep invoke this automatic cleanup. As you fast or sleep or both, your cells begin the process of looking for something to burn for energy. Inside your cells are lots of leftover "debris" that can be used for energy. This is the process of autophagy, and it happens when you fast and allows you to get rid of all that intracellular junk. It is actually an important biological process that keeps your cells healthy and vibrant while removing cell products that are not only unnecessary but potentially harmful if not "swept away."

You are both cleaning up your cells and using that cleanup as an energy source.

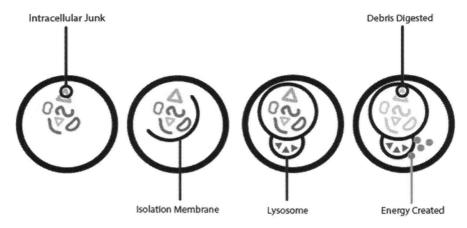

AMP-K signals Intracellular Junk / Debris Digested / Isolation Membrane / Lysosome / Energy Created

AMP-K

Fasting and exercise amplify AMP-K (adenosine monophosphate-activated protein kinase), an enzyme that increases energy molecules in a variety of ways shown by the following diagram. AMP-K signals your body to burn glucose, not store it as fat. It stimulates the uptake of glucose by muscle cells, inhibits the creation of fatty acids and cholesterol, and increases fatty acid utilization. It has some additional benefits of stimulating the creation of more mitochondria (the cell's energy factories), and it encourages the activation of antioxidant activity that suppresses chronic inflammation — the root of nearly all complex chronic illnesses. When AMP-K is active, it increases insulin sensitivity, which is so often lacking for those with obesity, diabetes, or metabolic syndrome. AMP-K is more activated during youth and less so as you age. In youth, it protects you from gaining fat weight and is protective against obesity and diabetes. When it wanes later in life, that protective effect diminishes. However, you can encourage this cellular "master switch" into activity because its most potent activator is exercise, with fasting synergistically adding to that effect.

Active AMP-K

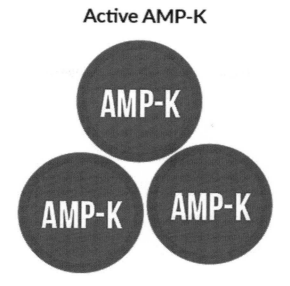

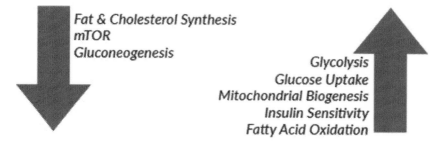

Fat & Cholesterol Synthesis
mTOR
Gluconeogenesis

Glycolysis
Glucose Uptake
Mitochondrial Biogenesis
Insulin Sensitivity
Fatty Acid Oxidation

Lipoprotein Lipase

What else can affect fat burning? Lipoprotein lipase (LL) is an enzyme that burns fat and is generated by changes in position. Your early morning HIIT exercise will rapidly increase lipoprotein lipase, but so will less intense activities. Get up from your chair periodically throughout the day and do some squats or jumping jacks or maybe climb up a few flights of stairs and back. Sitting all day is bad for your health in many ways, and this is one more reason to move about regularly. Remember, *"Sitting is the new smoking."* We are not talking about vigorous exercise here, just regular movement throughout the day. Break the cycle of sitting for a meal, sitting while driving to work, sitting at a desk all day, sitting while driving back home, sitting while eating dinner, and then sitting some more to watch television. Get up and move — frequently.

If you simply do not like the term "fasting," then restate it as "time-restricted eating." You are keeping your eating time to the hours between 10 a.m. and 7 p.m. or noon to 8 p.m.

The message is clear — fasting has many benefits for your body, and when added to an exercise regimen, it has real power to help you maintain wellness and health.

Here are more benefits of fasting for twelve to fifteen hours each day:

- Fasting increases glycolysis, meaning more sugar-burning.

- Fasting uses up the stored glycogen (glucose) in the liver.

- Fasting improves your sensitivity to insulin and reverses insulin resistance.

- Fasting increases the number of mitochondria in the cells, or the energy-burning generators.

- Fasting helps you burn fat and decrease cholesterol synthesis.

- Fasting increases autophagy and sweeps up trash from your cells.

- Fasting slows down the mTOR-aging pathway (more about this later).

To summarize, a growing body of evidence shows that prolonged overnight fasting (a.k.a. time-restricted eating) is particularly effective for losing weight. Paired with a low carbohydrate diet and HIIT, fasting will help you become an effective fat-burning machine. *What* you eat is obviously important, but *when* you eat is equally critical. Even healthy foods after your evening meal can be unhealthy.

Remember, this is more than just burning off your "overfat." You will be enhancing your overall health.

Another term that is apropos is "circadian rhythm fasting" since the fasting time relates to the body's natural time of quiet. When this is combined with a quality diet and regular exercise, it improves health overall and reduces weight and overfat. It is an approach that research indicates is especially effective for those with type 2 diabetes mellitus or metabolic syndrome.

Do not let the term "fasting" deter you. We are not talking about some lengthy process or special diet with juices. It simply means not eating between dinner and breakfast, preferably a dinner (or a supper if your main meal is at midday) finished early in the evening and a breakfast delayed sufficiently to allow for twelve but preferably fifteen hours without any food intake other than water, coffee or tea — without sugar, of course.

A few final thoughts: Fasting/time-restricted eating is not a binge-and-purge program. It is a way to develop a new and possibly different relationship with your food. Do not get obsessed. There is no need to feel stressed. Remember, you should be sleeping during most of the fasting time.

If you would like to read more about intermittent fasting, check out the article in the reference noted here.[5] Or watch the first part of the video in this reference.[6]

* * *

When you do get up to move a bit, here is a simple but valuable exercise to affect how you look and feel. Exercise your transversus abdominous (TA) muscle, the deep muscle that gives your abdomen structure by holding in your belly. The exercise is simple. Pull in your navel and hold it for five seconds. Do not hold your breath and keep breathing. Let the muscle go and repeat ten times. If you do this periodically throughout the day, you may be pleasantly surprised at the reduction of your abdominal girth within three to six weeks. This will help your posture as well. Once you have mastered this standing, exercise the TA while squatting. You probably were told that doing sit-ups or crunches would be the best exercise for your belly and give you "washboard abs." It is certainly valuable to strengthen those muscles called rectus abdominous, but it is the TA that will impact your girth, posture and appearance, not the rectus. Go ahead and work on your washboard muscles if you want but do the TA exercise for your girth and posture.

BOOM! Week #4 Program

- Try time-restricted eating or intermittent fasting between 10 a.m. and 7 p.m. Either term is fine, and you will find that it is easier than you think.

- Use a food diary. Consider using the MyFitnessPal app.

- Eat in a low glycemic fashion.

- If you have not done so yet, try to go two weeks with a total carbohydrate count less than 50-60 grams per day.

- Do not just think it, say it out loud: "I am not going to eat that donut."

- Do your HIIT workout after your overnight fast, except for hydrating with coffee, water, or tea, but no sugar.

- Do not eat for at least two hours after HIIT.

- Do HIIT workouts twice per week.

- Do your regular aerobic exercise, such as a thirty-minute walk, four other days of the week.

- Do your resistance exercises twice per week, preferably on the same days as HIIT.

- Move! Get up from your desk every hour, do some squats, pull your belly in (the TA exercise), and get 7,500 to 10,000 steps.

- Notice how much better you feel!

Not eating anything after supper proved another challenge for Jennifer. She usually had a "little something" shortly before bed. Perhaps a small dish of ice cream or some cheese. Call it comforting. However, she found this was a fairly easy thing to do without.

CHAPTER 6: THE VALUE OF FASTING FOR HEALTH AND LONGEVITY

"Almost everything will work again if you unplug it for a few minutes ... including you." - Anne Lamott

Calorie Reduction and Fasting as Health Aids

Reconsider what you eat and reduce the carbohydrates that you eat. Specifically, this means to reduce dramatically the amount of sugar and refined white flour in your diet. Americans tend to eat an average of 154 pounds of added sugar per year, based on an average of all the sugar manufactured and sold in the U.S. per year. The actual amount consumed per person is undoubtedly less, and some estimates say about 75 pounds per year. Whether it is 75 or another number up to 154 does not matter — what does matter that it is a tremendous amount of sugar. Another way to look at it is how many five-pound bags of sugar that would be sitting on your kitchen table — thirty. That is a lot. If you are a two-person family, that means sixty bags of sugar, and if you are a four-person family, that is 120 bags of sugar being eaten during the course of a year. Yikes.

Of course, if you do not eat that much sugar (about a half-pound per day or about 225 grams), then someone else must be eating even more than 154 pounds a year to make it an average! Is it possible that there is that much sugar in your diet? Recall that the average adult male should have no more than about 37 grams of sugar a day and a woman no more than about 25 grams a day. One can of soda has about 39 grams of sugar in it, and some bottles have much more. Many people do not have a single 12-ounce can per day but rather multiple cans throughout the day or even a "Big Gulp" cup of soda, which makes the consumption of sugar go up quite dramatically. Add to this the sugar that gets added to coffee or tea or sweetened iced tea (a well-known bottled iced tea has 65 grams of sugar in a small bottle!), as well as the sugar that is in ice cream and the sugar that is in many fruit yogurts, and you begin to see that it is pretty easy to eat that amount of sugar. How about that donut mid-morning or the pastry mid-afternoon? Or that snack that comes out of the refrigerator around 10 o'clock at night? All of these tend to have sugar in them, and since it is much more than you need for energy purposes, that sugar goes right to your belly and creates fat.

The other thing that creates fat is white flour. Recall again that white flour is digested in your mouth and intestine into sugar. Obviously, white flour is the basic ingredient in breads, cakes, pies, cookies, pasta and, yes, even pizza. We need to reduce the amount of these carbohydrates that come with few nutrients in them.

While eating, it would not be a bad idea to fit food consumption into a shorter window. What is a shorter window? Years ago, the farmer came inside to have a mid-morning "break-fast" and then had the main meal or dinner at 12 or 1 o'clock. Supper was a smaller, lighter meal finished fairly early. It was very unusual in those times to have snacks as we tend to do today. They did not take a coffee break in the morning and afternoon, and they did not have that late-night trip to the refrigerator.

So that shorter window for you might mean having a later breakfast and a somewhat earlier supper with the extra advice to have your main meal during the middle of the day so it can be well digested long before it is time for bed.

Why is it important to not eat after supper and until a later breakfast? We will be a bit repetitive here because it is so important that you understand the rationale for time-restricted eating/overnight prolonged fasting. The answer is that when we eat, particularly carbohydrates, the sugar from them is taken to our various cells in our body and used for energy. But once there is no need for any more sugar, the remainder gets stored in the liver in a temporary form called glycogen. Glycogen can be readily converted back into glucose (sugar) to circulate in the bloodstream and into the cells that need it. But if the glycogen storage area gets filled, added ingested glucose is converted from sugar into fat for either storage in the liver or in the fat cells, especially the fat cells in the belly. Not eating after supper until mid-morning the next day gives an opportunity for the glycogen in the liver to be converted back to glucose and used by the cells, so that by tomorrow morning, the glycogen has been used up and it is time to restart the filling process. While that is happening overnight, our body starts to make growth hormone or human growth hormone (HGH). When we were kids, this helped us grow. HGH has many other important metabolic functions, including

Decline of HGH with Age

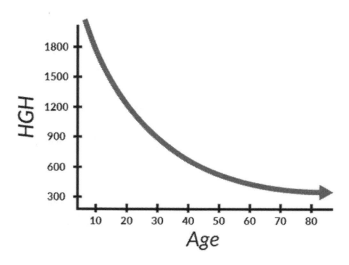

maintaining muscle mass, but HGH levels decline dramatically with age.

You make more growth hormone when your body has depleted its glycogen stores, when insulin levels are low and when you are asleep. It is good to have that growth hormone increase, but it will drop down as soon as your sugar levels go up and insulin levels go up after eating a breakfast of cereals or carbohydrates. Delaying breakfast an hour or two gives some extra time for that sleep and exercise-induced increase in growth hormone to have a beneficial effect.

This concept raises an important question: Is when you eat as important as how much you eat? There are four approaches, perhaps more, to improving health through either eating less food or adjusting the time of eating.

Calorie Restriction

The first involves calorie restriction, which we all know is usually called dieting. In such an approach, you usually reduce the number of calories consumed each day by 10 to 40 percent. There are so many different types of diets with all sorts of different names. It is a huge business with books, TV shows and organizations all there to help you lose weight (and your dollars). What we do know is that most of these work for a while, but then the pounds come back. An obvious question: Is there more to decreasing calories? It is known that in mice and rats, reducing the number of calories improves metabolism, increases lifespan, and improves health. Reducing calories by about 30 to 40 percent dramatically increases the lifespan of a mouse. It also improves their immunity and lowers cancer incidence, but if that calorie restriction is increased slightly past 50 percent of normal, longevity declines quite rapidly.

Animal Life Span
as a Result of Restricting Calories

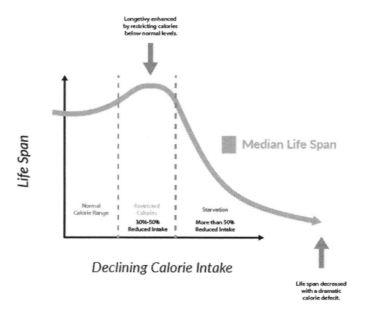

In human studies, it is clear that restricting calories improves metabolism and health, but it is hard in a human situation to demonstrate that lifespan improves. At the same time, there is some anecdotal evidence. Consider the five Blue Zones. In Okinawa, Japan, for example, we know that the individuals who live there have a fairly sparse diet, especially during World War II and before that in the Depression. Even after the war, they had a restricted diet for many years, and today there is a large percentage of centenarians on Okinawa who lived through that Depression and those post-war years.

Time-Restricted Eating

Time-restricted eating recommends eating the same number of calories and the same types of foods as usual but simply limiting when the food is eaten. It also defines a window during the day, usually between four and twelve hours, in which to eat. The question is: Will the benefits of calorie restriction or calorie reduction be met just as well by adjusting the time of eating, and conversely, by the amount of time fasting? It is a fascinating concept. You do not have to eat less; you simply have to eat over a limited span of time and perhaps there will be an improvement in health. An option from the usual pattern of eating, for example, might be to fast for about fifteen hours from 7 p.m. at night after finishing supper until the next morning at 10 a.m. Said another way, time-restricted eating means you will eat all of your food between 10 a.m. and 7 p.m. during a nine-hour period.

What does this do? Basically, it protects against the metabolic consequences of a Western diet. In animals, this leads to a reduction in weight, an increase in energy use, improved glucose control, lower insulin levels and reduced inflammation. These are all good.

During the day, your cells are busy with energy expenditure. During nighttime sleep, the cells focus on maintenance, repair and rest. What is interesting is that the benefits of time-restricted eating come independent of the diet composition. It can be exactly the same diet, as in the case with the mice.

The key is the amount of time, not eating. It is also important when that window of time of eating occurs. It is best to eat the bulk of the calories mid-day and leave later in the day for a lower caloric intake. Said differently, sticking to our normal body circadian rhythm, both in time spent eating and the timing of eating, can be advantageous. In other words, we spend far too much time over the course of a day eating and eating late in the day shifts how our body tries to recover during the course of the night.

This window of fasting, meaning the time after the last meal of the day and before the first meal of the next day, is when our cells switch from their daytime cell growth and reproduction phase to a nighttime cell maintenance and repair phase. Just like it is time to put the car in the garage and leave the engine off for a while, we could say that the human body needs some time "off." Of course, our cells are still functioning, but now they can switch over to the repair and maintenance phase, which is important for the maintenance of health in each of our cells. So, in short, when you eat is perhaps just as important as how much you eat and what you eat.

Intermittent or Periodic Fasting

Instead of just fasting overnight or for a slightly longer period of time, what about a third possibility? Intermittent, or periodic, fasting occurs when you either partially or completely stop food intake, taking perhaps just water and some vitamins, and this could be done from one to several days. A wit once said that the one thing that Jesus, Mohammad, and the Buddha all agreed on was the value of fasting.

In our past, humans often went days, even weeks, without food. They had to worry about going out and hunting for food or finding nuts, berries, and seeds, and if they did not find those for some period of time, they still had to survive. Our bodies were built for that, and the fat around our belly, in particular, was used to carry us through those times of no food. Of course, today we have instant gratification when hungry and we have not just an occasional meal but a routine of at least three meals a day — probably six because so many people have that mid-morning break, an afternoon break and then a late evening repast.

The idea of intermittent fasting or periodic fasting is that, similar to overnight fasting, we can shift the energy use from growth and reproduction in our cells to maintenance, recycling and repair. This is very important for our cells, and so there is a true advantage in a period of fasting every day. The question is: Would longer fasting be valuable?

In rodents, intermittent fasting leads to less obesity, less cardiovascular disease, a reduction in blood pressure, a reduction in the onset of diabetes and a reduction in the onset of neurodegenerative diseases. In addition, it reduces the incidence of cancer, retards the growth of tumors and improves the effectiveness of cancer chemotherapy. Intermittent fasting can also improve immunity, increase autophagy and decrease inflammatory markers. Definitely, it is all very positive. But a mouse is often not the best model for how a human will respond to the same thing. It turns out there are only a few short-term human studies, but the ones that have

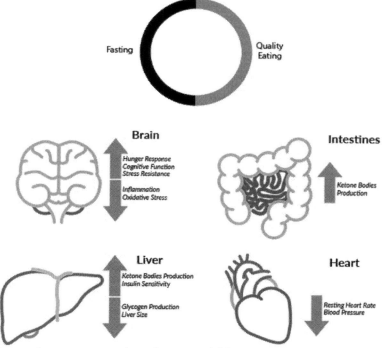

been done suggest that there could be reasonable weight loss of fat and better cardiometabolic health. Certainly, there are many anecdotal stories of how some type of fasting or another has improved a person's health or at least their sense of well-being.

Should you feast or should you famine? Neither is the right answer. You should eat a quality diet like the Mediterranean diet and do so moderately. For the BOOM program and beyond, we recommend you reduce total carbohydrates, especially sugar and white flour. We also recommend you fast after supper and at least until breakfast, preferably longer. On HIIT days, fast until about 10 or 11 a.m., or you may find you are okay until noon.

Fasting Mimicking Diet

There is a new concept out called the fasting mimicking diet. It offers a modest reduction in calorie intake and composition that seems to equate with fasting as far as the body is concerned. That is why it is called a "mimicking" diet. The composition is really the key here since it keeps the insulin levels from rising and, as a result, human growth hormone and other important chemicals can be at their peak value. The fasting mimicking diet was developed by scientists at the University of Southern California and funded by the National Institute of Aging. It has a lower carbohydrate level but a higher fat level and a moderate degree of protein. It is reduced in calories and includes such things as plant-based soups, herbal teas, energy bars (with very little sugar in them), various nut-based snacks and vitamin and mineral supplements.

Part of the idea here is that you do not need to feel like you are going to be "starved" during a period of fasting. Instead, there will be something to eat and you will feel satisfied if not exactly satiated. The concept of the fasting mimicking diet is to keep the glucose and insulin levels low, increase the production of ketones, improve the development of stem cells and limit inflammatory markers. In mice, researchers have been able to compare a standard diet to the fasting mimicking diet and show an improved immune system, increased longevity, lower cancer rates, improved cognitive measures and improved stem cells. These are all the measurements that you can accomplish with a period of fasting with water, minerals and vitamins.

There has also been a study using the fasting mimicking diet in humans. Considered a pilot study, it included nineteen individuals in good health who ate their standard diet and nineteen others also in good health who agreed to eat the fasting mimicking diet. They ate the diet for five days at the beginning of each month, followed by their standard diet for the rest of the month. This was repeated five times. Comparing the control individuals to those who ate the fasting mimicking diet, the researchers found a decrease in risk factors for aging, diabetes, cardiac disease, and cancer. Of course, five months is not enough time to see whether diseases themselves actually occur or whether lifespan would be increased, but they were certainly able to show a lot of positive benefits from the fasting mimicking diet. There is a caution here, of course. Animal models can be exciting, but they may not be a good predictor of what will happen in humans, and this one pilot human trial is not enough to say that this is "the thing to do."

Dr. Oken used the fasting mimicking diet himself and then with a group of twelve intrigued volunteer patients. His observations: All twelve completed the five days. He was not hungry but not satiated either, and the food was fine but boring by the end of the five days. He felt that he had more energy, his mental capacities were stronger, and these feelings lasted for a while after the end of the five days. In addition, he felt that he was less achy, which continued for months. About five months later, he did the diet again and had the same observations. We conclude this may be a strategy that can be helpful as we age. Moreover, since inflammatory markers decline using this approach, it may be helpful for patients with significant inflammation, repeated every two to three months until the inflammation improves clinically.

It is fair to summarize by saying that calorie restriction, time-restricted eating (a.k.a. the long overnight fast), intermittent or periodic fasting for five days each month, or the fasting mimicking diet used for five days each month all appear to be beneficial for health. The sum total of this is that when you eat appears to be as important as what you eat and how much you eat.[7]

***

Gratitude

Here is a suggestion that can help you sleep more soundly and generally enjoy life more fully. Each evening before bed, stop and think about something that was especially pleasurable today. It need not be something "big" or complex. Maybe you were out on your walk and saw a bright red cardinal against the snow. You watched him for a few moments and he flew away, but you found you were smiling. Now, lying in bed, bring up that image and the feeling you had at the time. Smile again. Better yet, write it down. Each day think of something different that happened that gave you a feeling of pleasure. Be grateful for the experience and write it down in a notebook. Do this every evening. It will not only give you a momentary smile and better sleep — you will be among those who live longer, have better health, and have a warmer outlook on life.

***

BOOM! Recap:

- Log your food. You eat more than you think.

- Try to keep your net carbohydrate count less than 50 grams per day. (Net carbs = Total carbs - fiber).

- If you are trying to reset your pleasure center, keep total carbs less than 50 for a week!

- Do the HIIT exercise fasting, except for hydrating with coffee, water, or tea.

- Try not to eat for at least two hours after exercise.

- Do two HIIT sessions each week.

- Do not just think it, say it out loud: "I am not going to eat that XXX."

- Move! Get up from your desk every hour, do some squats, pull your belly in, get 7,500 to 10,000 steps every day!

- Eat in a low glycemic fashion.

- Do some resistance (weight) exercises twice per week, preferably on the same day as the HIIT exercise.

- Be on fructose patrol! Have the right size serving of fruit, but be careful with dried fruit, which is full of fiber but also full of crystallized fructose.

- Your pleasure center is strong, but you are stronger, and you can beat it down by avoiding moderate to high glycemic carbs.

- Try prolonged overnight fasting, a.k.a. time-restricted eating. It is easier than you think. If you prefer, call it time-restricted eating with an eating window from 10 a.m. to 7 p.m.

- Recruit your TA. Pull that belly in!

- Do not drink your calories, and drink water when thirsty.

Jennifer was now "hooked" on prolonged overnight fasting. Skipping her long-held practice of a late-night ice cream snack was easy, and it comported with her efforts to reduce total carbs, especially sugar. She felt better. She was not hungry when she arose in the morning. Surprised initially, she was not famished after the HIIT workout and resistance training. Waiting until about 10 a.m. for a late breakfast was actually quite comfortable.

CHAPTER 7: MORE ON EXERCISE

"Practice puts brains in your muscles." - Sam Snead

> *"Lack of activity destroys the good condition of every human being, while movement and methodical physical exercise save it and preserve it." (Plato, about 400 BCE)*

A more modern statement was in *Time* magazine:

> *"… the most effective, potent way that we can improve quality of life and duration of life is exercise. The price is right too." (Oaklander, M., The New Science of Exercise, Time Health, Sept 12, 2016)*

What both of these say is exercise will lengthen your life and prevent disease, which is a good return on investment.

We are a sedentary population. We go from bed to breakfast chair, to car, to desk, to car, to chair for dinner, to sofa for TV and finally to sleep. This is completely different from our recent forebearers who were up and about nearly all day long. It is also not at all the pattern of the centenarians in the five Blue Zones.

There is good experimental evidence regarding the critical role of exercise in maintaining good health. For example, when a group of mice with genetics that caused them to age prematurely were divided into two groups, with one group that exercised three times per week and one group that was sedentary, the results were striking. At the end of five months, the sedentary mice were shriveled and had less functional hearts, coarse and gray fur, thinned skin and hearing loss. The mice that exercised were healthy, indeed as healthy as normal mice, and despite their genetic predisposition to aging rapidly, they did not. This is another example that genetics need not be destiny.

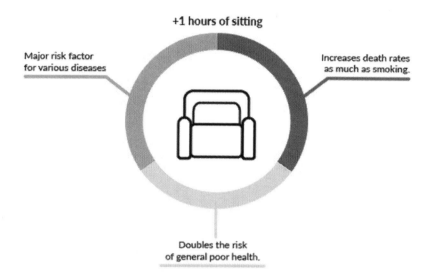

+1 hours of sitting

Major risk factor
for various diseases

Increases death rates
as much as smoking.

Doubles the risk
of general poor health.

"Sitting is the new smoking." Sitting for long periods (more than one hour) is a major risk factor for various diseases, poor health overall and an earlier death. Chronic sitting increases death rates as much as smoking! Inactivity doubles the risk of general poor health. Just standing up rapidly activates the body systems that control blood sugar, cholesterol, and triglycerides. Exercise improves the cells' ability to respond to insulin, whereas sitting increases the propensity toward insulin resistance (and later diabetes). In essence, the human body needs to move for its cellular and metabolic processes to work normally. Sitting has the opposite effect.

It is well known that exercise is valuable to heart health, reduces blood pressure, strengthens and preserves muscle size and strength, reduces blood sugar and reduces body fat. It also preserves and amplifies brain function and size. In short,

"If it were a drug, exercise would be considered a miracle drug for health preservation." (Austad, S, A Young Field about Growing Older: Six Ways Research Is Changing How We Age, Huffington Post, October 12, 2016)

Only a small proportion of Americans get the recommended levels of exercise per week — 150 minutes of aerobic exercise (thirty minutes five days per week) plus resistance exercises two or three times each week. What is also important is not only to schedule some time each day, although that is clearly advisable, but also to get up and move about at least every hour for five to ten minutes all day long. Remember that exercise improves all body functions, not just muscles. For example, it benefits the structure and function of the brain, skin, heart, lungs, and even eyes — every part of the body.

You already know that exercise has been well documented to prevent the most important age prevalent diseases such as heart and lung disease, cancer, dementia, and diabetes. This reduction in prevalence is "dose dependent," which means the more exercise you do (up to a point), the less the disease rate. Too much exercise is not healthy either, but most individuals will never get to the "too much" level.

At the other end, the question remains: Is there a lower limit below which exercise is of no particular value? The answer is probably "no." It is clear that even short bouts of activity are valuable. That said, it is certainly best to obtain the recommended intervals. Less is still valuable, but more is definitely much better.

"Physical activity is one of the best modifiable factors for the prevention of noncommunicable disease and mortality." (Eijsvogels, T, Journal of the Amer Med Assoc, 2015)

Here are the basics that everyone should follow: Start with aerobic exercise for thirty minutes five or six days per week. The aerobic exercise can be something as simple as walking at a reasonably brisk pace for thirty minutes. If you have a fitness monitor, try to achieve at least 7,500 steps per day. More would be even better, and some set their step goals at 10,000. Do not sit for long. Instead, stand up at least every hour, or more often if possible. Move about before sitting again. Perhaps you can set up your desk so you can work standing up.

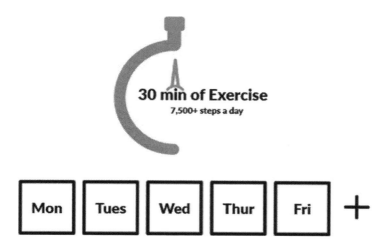

30 min of Exercise
7,500+ steps a day

| Mon | Tues | Wed | Thur | Fri | + |

With the BOOM program, you also now know that doing HIIT twice per week provides major added benefits, as does muscle resistance exercises twice per week. Each needs to be done to recruit the white fibers, which will help your muscles develop appropriately and release more growth hormone, a chemical that benefits many metabolic processes in the body. So, keep at it and remember the advantages of overnight fasting and waiting to eat for a few hours beyond your HIIT workout.

Start out slowly — there is no need to create sore muscles. Find a setting that feels appropriate for your needs and personality. Although most people find exercise stimulating and relaxing, it may not seem that way at first, and you may face an emotional barrier that needs to be overcome. A personal trainer might be valuable, especially at first. He or she can give you good advice and "keep you accountable" in a nonjudgmental manner. Remember, getting started now will lead to benefits that compound over time, just as a monetary investment for retirement compounds greatly over the years.

Consider taking a nice walk early in the morning or in the evening, preferably in a natural setting, but wherever is better than not. Many cultures emphasize the value of a contemplative walk, where you are alone with your thoughts and your observations of the world around you without focusing on the toils and concerns of the day. "Slowing down" can be restful, but more importantly, it can be an opportunity to "recharge." The stoics aimed to develop the inner life and found this type of walking enabled them to focus on their unconscious thoughts. Seneca said, "We should take wandering outdoor walks, so that the mind might be nourished and refreshed by the open air and deep breathing." Buddhism prioritizes walking as one of the four meditative positions. Buddhism also encourages moving the body to relax the mind, breathing with the pace of walking, and then looking for calm. Plus, creativity increases after a nice walk. Most walkers know that their mood heightens. The Japanese speak of "forest bathing" and the value of being in nature and away from the turmoil of day-to-day life. There is some science to this. Interestingly, walking beats running in reducing blood pressure, cholesterol, and the risk of heart disease.[8]

It is worth repeating that sitting is unhealthy. Get up. Move around. "*Sitting is the new smoking.*" Do not let it get you.

* * *

Let us reconsider growth hormone in more detail. It is a protein hormone created in the pituitary gland in the brain that impacts not only growth but many metabolic processes in the body. When growth hormone is secreted by the pituitary, it circulates in the blood and then binds to the surface of various target cells. Growth hormone stimulates the creation of proteins by increasing the uptake of amino acids from the bloodstream into targeted cells and then increasing the synthesis of actual proteins while decreasing the oxidation (breakdown) of proteins in the cell. In fat cells, growth hormone stimulates the breakdown of fats (triglycerides) into fatty acids and at the same time increases oxidation of fats in the fat cells, especially in the belly. Growth hormone helps to maintain the level of glucose in the blood in a fairly constant range. It inhibits the action of insulin to stimulate the uptake of glucose into various cells, and concurrently it stimulates the conversion of glycogen to glucose in the liver

Growth hormone production by the pituitary is greatest in adolescents during puberty when growth spurts occur. Over time, growth hormone levels continue to decline, and this impacts the aging process, including a decrease in lean body mass, an increase in fat mass and a decrease in bone density. This diminishment can lead to frailty, along with muscle wasting, abdominal obesity, fracture tendency and disrupted sleep. By recognizing these abnormalities as related, at least in part, to low levels of growth hormone, some scientists have attempted to reverse it with growth hormone injections. Results have been equivocal at best with some increase in lean body mass, muscle mass, decreased fat and improved skin turgor but with some distinct unwanted side effects. We do not recommend getting injections unless there is a distinct medical reason. Instead, boost your GH level with fasting and exercise.

Growth hormone is a major regulator of carbohydrate and lipid metabolism through its direct effects and its indirect effects with insulin-like growth factor-1, or IGF-1. Growth hormone tells fat cells to break down triglycerides, the compound that we call fat. At the same time, it prevents the fat cells from taking up new fatty acids circulating in the bloodstream. Its indirect effects come from stimulating the liver to produce and release IGF-1. In turn, IGF-1 stimulates bone growth, muscle growth and the development of new muscle cells.

Growth hormone is primarily produced during deep sleep, but output increases with exercise, especially vigorous exercise. When seven men with moderate exercise training did vigorous exercise, their growth hormone levels rose. Each man ate a limited breakfast at 6 a.m. and did not exercise one week, then exercised at 10 a.m., 11:30 a.m. and 1 p.m., and in the next week, at 10 a.m., 2 p.m. and 6 p.m. Blood was drawn every ten minutes to measure growth hormone levels.

This graphic shows how exercise drove up growth hormone levels, which then dropped quickly but persisted at levels above the control week (with no exercise) for about two hours.

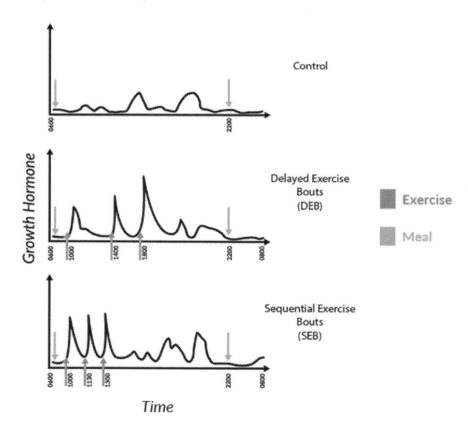

With a few hours of delay between vigorous exercise cycles, the levels of growth hormone rose further with each cycle. The growth hormone levels with subsequent sleep were normal.[9]

It is from studies like this that we advocate you do the HIIT exercises on a twice weekly schedule to both maximize the strength building of your muscle and the output of growth hormone, and as a result, promote bone density, fat metabolism, blood sugar control and lean body mass and muscle.

Having a desk job meant that Jennifer sat a good part of the day. Her office was on the fourth floor, so she started climbing the stairs rather than taking the elevator. Then she set her phone to vibrate every hour to remind her to stand up and move about for a few minutes. Sometimes she went back to the staircase and walked down a floor or two and then back up. After a while, she realized that she was more alert as she worked.

CHAPTER 8: FREAKING FRUCTOSE

"Very simply, we subsidize high-fructose corn syrup in this country, but not carrots. While the Surgeon General is raising alarms over the epidemic of obesity, the President is signing farm bills designed to keep the river of cheap corn flowing, guaranteeing that the cheapest calories in the supermarket will continue to be the unhealthiest." - Michael Pollan

Fructose

Fructose is a five-carbon sugar found in vegetables and fruit but not in a concentrated form. Consuming low levels of fructose on a daily basis is not unhealthy. However, our modern diet is overly abundant with excessive concentrated fructose. Concentrated fructose is used as a sweetener, usually derived from corn, and is called high fructose corn syrup (HFCS). It is used in thousands of food products and soft drinks.

Excessive fructose consumption causes metabolic damage and triggers the early stages of diabetes and heart disease. It also contributes to the development of insulin resistance, obesity, high blood pressure, elevated triglycerides, and low-density lipoprotein.

If you ingest fructose only from fruits and vegetables, as most people did a century ago, you will consume about 15 grams per day. More recently, however, the average American consumes greater than *60 grams per day or 48 pounds per year,*[1] largely from processed foods and sweetened drinks, which means that a remarkably high 10 percent of calories in the American diet comes from fructose.

Fructose is harmful in large doses. In vegetables and fruits, it is mixed with fiber, vitamins, minerals, enzymes, and beneficial phytonutrients. These accompanying nutrients moderate the negative metabolic effects of fructose.

Today, 55 percent of sweeteners used in food and beverage manufacturing is high fructose corn syrup. The primary fructose source of calories in America is soda. To be exact, HFCS is a mix of fructose and glucose but our attention here is on the fructose. Food and beverage manufacturers began switching their sweeteners from sucrose (table sugar) to high fructose corn syrup in the 1970s. It is much less expensive and about 20 percent sweeter than table sugar. It is estimated that about one-quarter of the calories consumed by Americans is in the form of added sugars, and most of that is HFCS.

As we have noted previously, the average Westerner consumes a staggering 75-154 *pounds* of added sugar each year, with much of that being high fructose corn syrup. Does 154 pounds sound impossible? It does until you stop and think about it. It means that each day the average consumption is one-half pound, or about 225 grams. That one twelve-ounce can of soda has 39 grams, and most people who drink soda have multiple sodas per day, often in even larger sizes. Add in some pasta, pizza, bread, gravy, and a few cookies, and it adds up quickly.

Fructose is absorbed differently than glucose. Glucose transits across the intestinal cell smoothly and quickly. Fructose does not. It follows a different route, and if one eats a high fructose meal, it cannot all be transported immediately. That remaining sugar in the gut can feed

---

[1] A reference from the Illinois Farm Bureau in 2009 indicated 36 pounds per year; whichever, it is a lot!

bacteria that should not normally be in large numbers, so they multiply rapidly in the small intestine, which is a syndrome known as small intestinal bacterial overgrowth (SIBO). The fructose fermentation process by the bacteria leads to gas formation, bloating and discomfort. SIBO is discussed in more detail later.

Your body metabolizes fructose in a much different way than glucose. Recall that glucose goes directly to the cells of the muscle, brain, and other organs and is used as the major energy source, which allows a muscle to contract. Glucose absorbed from a meal that is not immediately needed is sent to the liver and stored as glycogen until called upon. If there is still more glucose absorbed from the gut than the body needs for energy and is more than the liver can store, the remainder is sent to fat cells where it is converted to fat or is stored in the liver as fat.

The entire burden of fructose metabolism falls on the liver. The biochemistry of fructose metabolism is complex. Fructose cannot be used directly by your cells for energy, so it is turned into liver glycogen, free fatty acids and triglycerides, which then get stored as fat. The fatty acids created during fructose metabolism accumulate as fat droplets in your liver. This contributes to the development of insulin resistance (the precursor to diabetes), various lipids circulating in the bloodstream and non-alcoholic fatty liver disease.

Consuming glucose, in general, does not produce much fat, but fructose does, perhaps by as much as 40 to 1. The metabolism of fructose by the liver creates a long list of by-products and toxins. Finally, and we will repeat this in the next chapter, glucose suppresses the hunger hormone ghrelin and stimulates leptin, thus reducing your sense of hunger. Fructose has no effect on ghrelin and interferes with your brain's communication with leptin, which contributes to over-eating.

Here are a few suggestions to limit fructose ingestion:

- Read labels. Do not consume products with high fructose corn syrup, including sodas, candy, pastries, cookies, cakes, pies, most packaged cereals, many prepared foods, yogurts, and iced tea.

- Avoid agave syrup since it is a highly processed sap that is almost all fructose.

- Use organic cane sugar and honey in moderation since both are about 50 percent fructose.

- Instead, use safe organic sweeteners such as stevia and erythritol (more later).

- Limit dried fruit, which is crystallized fructose and more calories than you think!

But do eat a few servings of fruit each day. They are vitally important to your health. Vary which fruits and choose multiple colors. The fructose in the fruit comes with many nutrients that your body needs.

Remember that the food manufacturing industry puts sweeteners in many foods but uses other terms that may not sound like "sugar." The industry is required to indicate sucrose as sugar on labels, but other sweeteners can simply be listed without you necessarily knowing that they are essentially sugars in one form or another. Look for them on labels before buying. Here is a list of commonly used sweeteners:

Agave nectar	Evaporated cane juice	Malt syrup
Brown sugar	Fructose	Maple syrup
Cane crystals	Fruit juice concentrates	Molasses
Cane sugar	Glucose	Raw sugar
Corn sweetener	High-fructose corn syrup	Sucrose
Corn syrup	Honey	Syrup

Crystalline fructose	Invert sugar	
Dextrose	Maltose	

A few final comments on sitting. Most people today sit for nearly 80 percent of their waking hours. When sitting for a short time, major changes occur in your body's metabolism. The cellular activity in your legs declines. Various critical enzymes like lipase drop precipitously. And the results? Sitters have about a 50 percent greater chance of dying of a heart attack. Sitters have double or triple the risk for heart disease, obesity, and diabetes.[10]

Unfortunately, you cannot make up for sitting all day with an hour at the gym. You need to stand up for at least a few minutes every hour. In one study, actors were recruited to live like our ancestors in the 1850s, meaning chopping wood, foraging for food, and doing other common activities of the time. Their movement was compared to a group of typical office workers. The 1850s group walked three to eight miles more per day.

Recommendation: Set a timer on your smartphone to be sure you do not get engrossed in a project and forget. Standing is just too important to forget.

BOOM! Week #5 Program

- Use your food diary every day.

- If you have not done so yet, try to go two weeks with your total carbohydrate count less than 50-60 grams per day. This will be a low glycemic diet.

- Plan to do the HIIT fasting, except for hydrating with coffee, water, or tea.

- Try not to eat for at least two hours after exercise.

- This combination of limited carbohydrates, HIIT and fasting during exercise will burn off fat.

- Prolonged overnight fasting is not as hard as you think. Think of it as restricted time eating if the idea of "fasting" is problematic for you. Remember, most of the "fasting" time is when you are asleep!

- It is best to do both HIIT sessions each week at the gym, but if that is impossible, consider the short-form home exercise mentioned in an earlier chapter.

- Do not think it, say it out loud: "I am not going to eat that donut."

- Move! Get up from your desk every hour, do some squats, pull your belly (TA) in, and get 10,000 steps every day.

- Continue doing resistance exercises with weights twice each week. Do this the same day as your HIIT exercise.

- Be on fructose patrol!

CHAPTER 9: YOUR PLEASURE CENTER

"The mind is everything." - Anonymous

Make your thoughts real by saying them out loud: "I am not going to eat that donut!" You control your pleasure center, and although it wants to, your pleasure center does not control you.

There is an area in our brain that directs our impulses to eat, which we will call the "pleasure center." We have trained it through our lifestyle. Our diet and activity level, as well as our emotions, play a role in modulating the pleasure center's effect on our behavior. The pleasure center's activity can be measured by functional magnetic resonance imaging (MRI) studies and positron emission tomography (PET) scans. Obese patients have been found to have overactive pleasure centers, but when they lose weight, the center is less active. Obesity is largely a brain-signaling problem. We evolved with a neural network hard-wired to avoid famine by our hunter-gatherer ancestors to feast on easy-to-store calories when available. But today, food is abundant, and food technology has increased the availability of easy-to-store calories, including moderate to high glycemic food. Basically, these are calorie dense but nutrient lite foods, which is the opposite of what your body needs. This is literally making us sick.

Obesity has been demonstrated to have a clear association with mortality. Comparing normal-weight individuals to obese individuals, people with obesity have a higher "all-cause mortality."[11] The National Institutes of Health indicates that obesity is now the major contributor and most common preventable cause of death, even exceeding tobacco-related deaths.[12] Obesity, per se, is usually not listed as a cause of death on death certificates, but the specific cause is usually one or more of the downstream diseases that obesity predisposes, especially heart disease, stroke, and to a lesser degree, cancer. Obesity also predisposes people to diabetes mellitus type 2, which itself is a predisposing risk factor for heart disease and stroke. As a result, we might speak of obesity as the number one killer in America!

Americans' life expectancy rose from about 35 years in 1850 to about 79 years in 2014. Then it began to fall, only slightly but consistently, for three years with a minimal rise in the fourth year. It is the result of the number of increasing deaths in mid-life from diseases of despair, such as suicide, alcohol, and drug overdose. Notably, it is also due to deaths from heart disease, which had fallen steadily for decades but began to rise. Why? The epidemic of obesity, followed by diabetes, is driven by the consumption of ultra-processed foods with high calories and limited nutrients along with little exercise, high stress, and poor sleep. We are looking toward a life expectancy catastrophe unless we each commit to changing our lifestyles.

Why do people continue to eat after their stomachs are full or even stuffed? The pleasure center overrides the rational thought center that tells you that you have had enough, and the more you override your rational thoughts, the stronger the pleasure center gets. This is how a habit is born and becomes stronger.

Our emotions, lifestyle, and diet affect our pleasure center. The pleasure center intensifies our cravings, often to a point that we cannot resist, and we strengthen the control of the pleasure center each time we succumb to its calling. The two main signaling hormones that are involved in this control are leptin and ghrelin.

Leptin tells us that we are "full" and is produced by fat cells. The more fat we carry, the more leptin we produce. However, in obese people, the high leptin levels begin to lose their inhibitory effect on hunger. This is called leptin resistance. Leptin overproduction by fat cells fails to cause that satiated feeling. This is a stumbling block for people with obesity since the signaling pathway does not work properly. The result is that the more obese you are, the harder it is to get lean and healthy. Obesity is a direct result of abnormal brain signaling due to a persistent and consistent diet filled with sugar, white flour, rice, corn, and potato.

The other important hormone is ghrelin, which is sometimes called the "hunger hormone." People who are given ghrelin experimentally become ravenous. Your body's level of ghrelin is influenced by many factors. Chronic lack of sleep increases this hormone, making you feel hungry when you really do not need to eat.

Insulin also plays a role in the level of ghrelin. The signaling system should work like this: You eat a sugary dessert, and insulin levels increase so the sugar in your blood can be taken to cells and used for energy. Eating sugar increases the production of leptin, which should decrease appetite and enhance fat storage. That sugar in the bloodstream also decreases the production of ghrelin, which regulates your food intake. Unfortunately, obesity, a lack of exercise, insulin resistance and poor dietary choices all cause the system to malfunction.

High fructose corn syrup (a mixture of fructose and glucose) is a cheaper form of sugar that is used in thousands of food products and soft drinks. Eating large amounts of fructose negatively affects metabolism since it is broken down in a different way than glucose, which is our primary fuel. Glucose suppresses the hunger hormone ghrelin and stimulates leptin, which suppresses your appetite. But fructose has no effect on ghrelin.

Fundamentally, what you are trying to do is break the addiction to sugar and sweets. If you want to control your sweet cravings, do not use artificial sweeteners since they perpetuate your desire for more sweets. Like any addiction, it can be difficult but definitely not impossible to overcome. Dealing with your pleasure center can be a challenge, but if you enlist willpower, you can do it and it will only become easier as time proceeds. Remember that willpower is the single most important habit for individual success.

Consider these important facts:

- Self-discipline has been shown to predict academic success more than intellectual talent.

- Willpower, with practice, can become automatic. It is a learnable skill.

- Unlike many skills, willpower does not remain constant.

- Willpower is like a muscle — the more practice, the stronger it gets.

- You are in control. Set goals, plan your day and see your health radically improve.

CHAPTER 10: STRESS

"Everything that irritates us about others can lead us to an understanding of ourselves." - Carl Jung

Jennifer had a job she enjoyed, a supportive boss who was not bothered by her coming in a bit late two days a week after her HIIT exercises and pleasant, cooperative coworkers. There was no clock to punch, and the expectation was to get the work done on time. Her problem was that, all too often, the boss assigned a new project with a short timeframe, and when the work was nearly done, he changed the requirements. This often meant late evenings because the client was coming tomorrow. She felt if she only had better instructions up front, she could do better work and always have it ready on time. What would he think if she told him he was causing stress to her and his other employees?

We have discussed diet and exercise, so now let us move to the third pillar of health — stress.

Chronic stress is underappreciated as a serious and common cause of inflammation, which is the root of nearly all chronic illnesses such as heart disease, arthritis, anxiety, and Alzheimer's, as well as many acute ones such as the common cold. Chronic stress is like a fire that has died down but is still smoldering quietly under the ashes — it is ready to burn widely if stoked. During that quiescent phase, it continually emits chemicals that aggravate inflammation. You will not even feel it happening, but it is there, and it occurs all day, every day. So, getting stress under control is absolutely critical to good health and wellness.

Hans Selye, MD, the physician who gave us the term "stress," has suggested, "The modern physician should know as much about emotions and thoughts as about disease symptoms and drugs. This approach would appear to hold more promise of cure than anything medicine has given us to date." There is a lot of truth here, but physicians (like all of us) do not pay it the attention that we should. We want you to focus on stress so you can get it under control and improve your life going forward.

Chronic stress releases epinephrine (adrenaline), cortisol and multiple other chemicals in a low and steady state, which is an unnatural condition. These are chemicals designed to alter body chemistry acutely to respond to an immediate danger like a truck careening toward you. You cannot fight it, so you must take flight — immediately. We have all felt the rapid heart rate and other symptoms of this fight-or-flight response. With chronic stress, the low but elevated epinephrine levels lead to an increase in heart rate, respiratory rate, and blood pressure, which can predispose to heart attacks, kidney damage and strokes. Elevated cortisol raises blood glucose, converts fats and carbohydrates to energy, elevates appetite and abdominal weight gain (which is a risk factor for cardiovascular disease), depresses the immune system (which leads to more infections) and disrupts sleep patterns (which contributes to poor concentration, injury and illness). Asthma attacks can increase in frequency and severity due to stress, and emotions can swing widely with anxiety and depression. Chronic stress adversely affects bone mineral density, which predisposes to osteoporosis, and it adversely affects cognitive function with memory impairment and reduced executive control. Chronic stress speeds up the aging process. In short, the result of chronic stress is clearly detrimental to good health and longevity.

Stress is a part of life and seems to intrude more and more. You cannot easily escape from all stressful situations, so you need to learn how to manage them. There are many ways to combat chronic stress. High on the list are a good diet and regular exercise. We suggest you try to always eat in a pleasant setting, preferably with some friends or coworkers. At home with family, dinner time should be with the whole family around the table as a daily time to be together and relax over good food. Actively think about the foods you are eating, including their appearance, taste, and smell. Chew slowly. This is a good way to change your eating patterns for the better.[13]

You may find yourself feeling much better after a moderately intense workout or even just after a pleasant walk in the woods where you enjoy nature all around you. Exercise is an effective way to reduce the impact of chronic stress.

Meditation is a great way to reduce stress, too. A simplified technique has been developed by Dr. Herbert Benson, a noted Harvard cardiologist in Boston. He calls it "the relaxation response." Fundamentally, it invites you to close your eyes, breathe slowly and deeply, and say a word or phrase silently to yourself repeatedly while exhaling. Your sense of ease will develop quickly, blood pressure will fall, and heart rate will fall. You can even do this with your eyes open in the checkout lane in the supermarket — but not while driving the car![14]

Yoga is another excellent way to reduce chronic stress while at the same time giving your muscles and tendons a good stretch. So is Tai Chi, or a slow-moving Chinese martial art that many people do every morning before anything else.

Also consider coherent breathing, biofeedback, acupuncture, and massage. Each can be greatly beneficial. The right music can be soothing as well, which can be played before bedtime to begin the relaxation process.

These are all ways to reduce ongoing stress. The other side of the equation is to limit the onset of stress. Imagine you have a difficult situation at work — can you encourage a change, or is it not possible? If the former, work on that, but if the latter and the stress is severe, maybe you need to look for a new position. Maybe you are too quick to say "yes" when asked by friends or clubs to take on a new role, project, or volunteer position. Of course, you want to help with your son's Boy Scout overnight, but if you do, then something else needs to go. Prioritize your time, and do not let it and you become overburdened. Learning to say "no" can be a huge help. You will quickly thank yourself. Remember, this is about your health, and preserving it is not selfish but vital.

Too much time on social media, emails at all hours, and other technology-heavy activities can have a negative impact on your health, according to a number of new studies. Frequent "multi-tasking" can lead to stress, anxiety and perhaps depression.[15] One study even used brain imaging to show a reduction in part of the brain. Of course, this is not proof that heavy involvement with multi-tasking leads to brain changes. Nevertheless, we suggest you think carefully about how much time you spend flitting back and forth with one thing or another, especially social media and emails. It's better to stick with a task, complete as much as you can and then move on.

Dr. Oken writes a newsletter for his patients each quarter. Here is an edited version of one about stress:[16]

"Anxiety, fear, and sadness are harmful to our health. These emotions cause all sorts of common and uncommon physical complaints. Negative thoughts disrupt our autonomic nervous system (palpitations, sleep abnormalities, chest pain, shortness of breath and hunger). Negative thoughts can squeeze our adrenal glands, causing changes in our cortisol and catecholamine levels. At the cellular level, it makes our T and B immune cells less functional, and at the molecular level, throws off the balance of our infection and age-fighting cytokines. Our mind becomes our foe instead of our friend.

Negative thoughts beget negative emotions and then we are unable to enjoy the present (a true gift). Our minds can take us to the future with worry, or the past, to beat ourselves up.

"You have a powerful mind; you probably are pretty good at making yourself feel bad, but the same neurophysiology can make you feel good. When we are happy, we feel better. When we are anxious, we may be fearful, irritable, and angry. Our emotions make us think a certain way and then our perceptions become our reality. Sometimes this is good and sometimes this is bad. We can lose sight that we control our thoughts and our thoughts control our emotions. This is particularly true if we are faced with a crisis: health, financial, family or friend issue. Our perception of the problem can get out of control and wreak havoc with our minds, which ultimately affects our physical and mental health. When we really get rolling, the dominoes are hard to stop, and before you know it, we feel like we are losing it. The excerpt below is from the book *10% Happier*, by Dan Harris.

"The Buddhists called this prapañca (pronounced pra-PUN-cha), which roughly translates to 'proliferation,' or 'the imperialistic tendency of mind.' That captured it beautifully, I thought: something happens, I worry, and that concern instantaneously colonizes my future."

Another idea to reduce stress is to actively distract yourself with a positive, enjoyable activity. Practice the concept of gratitude by taking a few moments each evening to consider at least one thing from the day that was positive and worthy of gratitude. It might be something simple such as a bird's song. The point is to finish the day on a positive note. Be aware if you are constantly telling yourself, "I should ..." These are basically negative thoughts and they build on each other. Laughter is a great way to relieve stress. Watch a TV comedy before bed or at any time of the day. Look for ways to convert a negative thought to something positive. What at first seems like a negative thought can, with some attention, often be converted.

Also, consider forgiveness. It is highly stressful to carry a grudge. Maybe you can resolve the underlying issue with the other person with some open discussion, either together or with a counselor. If that is not possible, then look for ways to "just let it go."

Here is more from Dr. Oken's newsletter:

"Take 5 minutes and play [some quieting music] and think of something pleasant. Notice how everything slows down, think of how fortunate and grateful you are for all that you have. And concentrate on your breathing; breathe through your nose, nice and slow. The music and breathing will allow you to take control of your mind. Experiment with your power. Think of a conflict or concern you have, and you probably will get some clarity to it. Perhaps you will realize that your worry just does not matter. Maybe you need to forgive someone, or even yourself, or maybe you need to just clear your mind. You may discover that your fears are just based on false evidence (F.E.A.R.= false evidence appearing real). Whatever it is, just breathe slowly and be in the moment. You may be surprised how you will feel and react.

"It takes work to quiet your mind. This is because many of us have unknowingly taught ourselves to be anxious. We have constructed neural pathways that are very fast and take us in lightning speed to panic, sadness and worry. But with concentration and perhaps meditation, or just thinking positive, we can reject those negative emotions. We can build super-fast neural pathways to take us to a calm, tranquil, constructive existence."

As a recap, look for ways to remove yourself from stressful situations or from too many obligations. Learn to say "no." Eat a healthy diet and do it mindfully with family, friends or coworkers. Make meals an event, not a chore. Move — any form of exercise will help reduce stress. Find your comfort zone with meditation, yoga, Tai Chi, acupuncture, massage, or a nice walk in the woods or on the beach. Consider doing coherent breathing. Keep thinking about gratitude each evening before bed and write down your thoughts. Use meditation, yoga, or Tai Chi to detach yourself from those recurring negative thoughts. Look for the positive in life and downplay the negative where possible. Having a good laugh can help. Forgive.

Jennifer was anxious but knew she should talk to her boss. The stress had gone on too long, and no amount of exercise or meditation could fully relieve it. She got up her courage, asked for some time and began by telling him he was very supportive and agreeable but there was one thing he could do to help them all. To her surprise, the boss was very approachable and seemed somewhat relieved to hear her. He said he knew he was often too quick to set parameters without fully thinking the project through. He promised to work on it and thanked her for talking to him. Maybe she and the others could help him by asking more questions when a new project came in, and perhaps they could all be sure the directions were clear. It seemed that he was as relieved as she was. A win-win.

BOOM! Recap:

- Try to keep your net carbohydrate count to less than 50 grams per day. Net carbs = total carbs - fiber grams. If you are trying to reset your pleasure center, keep total carbs less than 50 for a week!

- Log your food — you eat more than you think. Consider using MyFitnessPal.

- Come to BOOM in a fasting state, except for hydrating with coffee, water, or tea.

- Try not to eat for at least two hours after exercise.

- Try to get two HIIT sessions in each week. Check out the TabataPro app on your phone.

- Do not just think it, say it out loud: "I am not going to eat that XXX."

- Move! Get up from your desk every hour, do some squats, pull your belly in, and get 7,500 to 10,000 steps every day.

- Eat in a low glycemic fashion.

- Do some weight work twice per week.

- Be on fructose patrol! Have the right size serving of fruit and be careful with dried fruit, which is full of fiber but also full of crystallized fructose.

- Your pleasure center is strong, but you are stronger, and you can beat it down by avoiding moderate to high glycemic carbs.

- Try intermittent fasting, it is easier than you think. Eating window: 11 a.m. to 8 p.m.

- Recruit your TA. Pull that belly in!

- Eat and enjoy GOOD FAT.

- Eat healthy sources of protein. Use the Goldilocks principle — not too much and not too little.

- Eat lots of fiber.

- Eat one tablespoon of ground flax seed per day.

- Prebiotic foods include a lot of plant fiber, and the more, the better. Take 2,000 units of Vitamin D-3.

- Do not use artificial sweeteners.

- Be purposeful in taking vitamins and supplements. Know what you are taking and why.

- Ask your doctor if a baby aspirin is right for you.

- Dark chocolate? A healthy treat!

- Optimize your sleep. Get six-and-a-half to eight hours per night.

- Power naps can be good!

- Do not drink your calories, and drink when thirsty.

CHAPTER 11: WHAT HAS LED TO THE OBESITY EPIDEMIC IN AMERICA?

"You better cut the pizza in four pieces because I am not hungry enough to eat six." - Yogi Berra

The usual assumption is that the obesity epidemic is related to eating too many calories as compared to how many are burned each day — calories in must equal calories out. If you eat too many calories and don't use them, then you get fat. It seems pretty simple and basic. However, that it is not enough to explain the overfat epidemic. First, it implies that the individual must be at fault. You were told to diet and you did, but it did not work, or at least not consistently or for a prolonged period.

Maybe something is missing here. Throughout history, humans were not fat until about forty-five years ago. What has changed? One change is that we eat more — sometimes six meals (breakfast, morning coffee break, lunch, afternoon coffee break, dinner and late night snack) per day rather than three. But obesity doesn't come from the calories in those six meals alone, as important as they are. It is the rise and fall in insulin, pushing calories into fat cells in the liver and in the belly. And, as you have learned, insulin is overutilized, insulin sensitivity declines and it takes more insulin to achieve the same result. Called insulin resistance, this is a critical step toward metabolic syndrome and later to type 2 diabetes. This overworking of insulin also begins to exhaust the pancreas where insulin is manufactured.

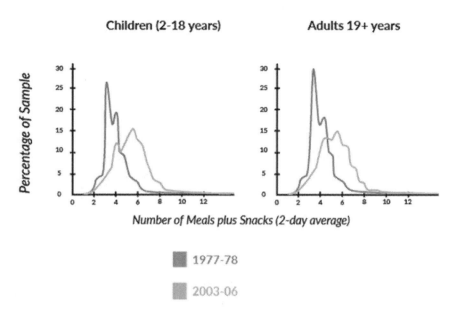

Children (2-18 years)   **Adults 19+ years**

Number of Meals plus Snacks (2-day average)

■ 1977-78

■ 2003-06

Unfortunately, the advice that people received from government agencies and other organizations during these past forty-five years has been to eat more meals and more carbohydrates and cut back on fat. Then came excessive use of refined white flour — in pasta, pizza, bread, cakes, pies, cookies, and pastries — and added sugar. Add to that the increased consumption of candy bars, sodas, ice cream, and more. Sugar consumption in America has increased rapidly to about 75-154 pounds per person per year, and white flour consumption is about 140 pounds per year per person. It sounds incredible and it is — and not at all healthy.

It is interesting that the U.S. Department of Agriculture food guidelines give recommendations for sensible eating, but its subsidies to farmers support the crops used in ultra-processed foods, including corn, wheat, and soybeans. Basically, your tax dollars encourage over-consumption of the wrong foods!

Yes, total calories "in" compared to total calories "out" is important, but it is not the whole story. All calories are not the same. You know intuitively that 100 calories from carrots must be much different than 100 calories from a candy bar. The overconsumption of carbohydrates multiple times each day prompts insulin to rise and put all of that carbohydrate in its place, either in the cells that need energy, the liver as fat or the fat cells in the abdomen. So, we might say that obesity is essentially a problem of hyperinsulinemia, or the overabundance of carbs that leads to an overuse of insulin, which then leads to insulin resistance and fat deposition.

Americans (and many people in other countries) are always looking for the culprit. Who did it? How can we hold him or her accountable? In the obesity epidemic, the culprit is usually said to be the person — he or she just does not have the willpower to resist. And he (or she) simply will not take the steps to cut back on calories and lose weight. The fat person is shunned and assumed to be guilty. It is one of the strongest biases ever. But maybe there is more to it, and maybe the person is not really the culprit.

We argue that the popular advice — to eat multiple meals per day, cut down on total fats and increase carbohydrates — is the initial culprit. Add to that the food processors that make and market fundamentally unhealthy products and most restaurants that prepare and market unhealthy meals and serve portion sizes way too large. No wonder we are an obese nation.

One culprit over the years has been saturated fats, including those found in dairy products. About forty years ago, the Department of Agriculture recommended a switch to no- or low-fat milk and dairy products as part of the effort to reduce the consumption of saturated fats. This advice, plus other advice to limit saturated fats, rapidly led to a massive shift in America to the use of low- and no-fat dairy products rather than whole fat dairy. Unfortunately, for whatever reason, today America has an epidemic of overweight, obesity, metabolic syndrome, diabetes, and an increasing incidence of cardiovascular disease. Was the dairy advice correct or not? A recent perspective article in the *Journal of the American Medical Association* [17] asked experts and suggested that the answer is simply not clear.

What is known about the health benefits or non-benefits is based on observational studies, which amount to correlations or associations rather than clear cause-and-effect data. Instead, randomized trials provide this type of data, where one group receives full-fat dairy and the other does not. Still, observational studies at least give directions for consideration. In the PURE study of more than 136,000 individuals between ages 35-70, a higher intake of dairy fat was actually associated with a lower risk of cardiovascular events and mortality. "Whole fat dairy seemed to be more protective than nonfat or low-fat dairy," the study authors wrote.

Another approach is to look at biomarkers by examining the blood content of three specific fatty acids recognized to be primarily derived from dairy products. It turns out that when sixteen such studies were pooled with 63,000 participants, those with higher levels of the dairy-associated fatty acids were less likely to develop diabetes during the time of the trial.

What about weight gain? It turns out there is no clear-cut evidence that full-fat dairy is more likely to lead to weight gain than low-fat or no-fat dairy consumption. An expert quoted in the article noted that there is no strong data to show that full-fat dairy leads to more weight, more cardiovascular disease, or more metabolic syndrome. Rather, observational studies suggest the opposite. Another expert who was interviewed suggested that the key is not to worry about any one ingredient in the diet but the overall dietary pattern. This makes good sense to us.

As you think about losing weight or simply improving your health, consider that the environment around you is not only unhelpful, it is outright against you. Society aims to overfeed you whether that is the local store, local restaurant, or food manufacturers. All create situations that undermine your best intentions. Portion sizes at restaurants have increased over the years. They know they put too much food on the plate, but they are afraid that if they do not, then you will go to their competition instead. We all know that fast food restaurants serve mostly unhealthy foods — the iconic bacon cheeseburger with fries and a large drink. But they market it well and since the double cheeseburger, large fries, and huge soda cost only a few pennies more than a regular size, why not supersize instead? Marketers tell you that the inherently unhealthy macaroni and cheese is really good, that yogurt with fruit (and sugar) is better than plain, or that prepackaged processed "all natural" breakfast bars are a good way to start the day. The sugar-coated cereal is at eye level where your kid sees it, but the plain yet healthy oatmeal is on the bottom shelf where neither of you can find it. In short, our economy conspires against our best efforts to eat "healthy and in moderation."

You can easily be sedentary since you can drive to work, use the drive-in window to get your breakfast, take the elevator up two floors, sit at your desk, then sit at your dinner table followed by time on the sofa watching TV. No need to stand or walk.

In addition, America makes you think that if you sleep more than five to six hours, you are cheating yourself and your company of time at work. You feel expected to check your emails before bed, encouraged to watch that high action movie late into the evening, and then watch the 11 o'clock news — filled only with the recent fires, murders, and other tragedies.

Life is full of elements that increase your anxiety. Those late-night emails make you stressed, yet if you don't check them, you feel equally stressed. What if the boss sent a request needed for tomorrow morning at 8 a.m.?

So, it seems the world is designed to defeat you. Your body tells you to eat sugars and carbs, avoid movement and spend more time on that sofa. Of course, you eat too much, walk too little, sleep way too little and are stressed out all the time. It is no surprise.

Restated, it is *not* your fault. You are not to blame for gaining weight, being less than healthy or being stressed. Do not blame yourself. It is not your personal failing. It is actually all of those out there who want to enrich themselves by pushing you to do yourself damage, although they would never admit it to themselves and certainly not to you. But at the same time, only you can make the change. Start by loving yourself as you are. Worry not about the future and be in the present. Question how you can make yourself better than you are and aim for who you want to be. You can change your life for the better, but it will be hard work because of the pressure around you. It's hard work but certainly possible.

It is also true that your body "set points" have changed as you gained weight. It has become the new "normal" and to change will be a real effort. Your microbiome has undoubtedly changed, and it takes a long time to work it back to where it was years ago.

* * *

Coherent Breathing

Coherent breathing, which is another technique to help you reduce stress and improve health, is not well-known, but it can be especially helpful to balance your internal signaling systems that are "revved up" from chronic stress. When you are stressed, your sympathetic nervous system is ratcheted up, and the parasympathetic system is reduced. Think of the sympathetic system as the active one and the parasympathetic as the relaxed one. The two systems are interconnected, and when one is more active, the other is less active.

Both are "autonomic," meaning they are not under voluntary control in the same way that you can control certain muscles or your eyes.

As a general rule for organs that respond primarily to the autonomic system, you cannot voluntarily control or manipulate them. You cannot control the rate of your heartbeat, the process of your digestion, how your hormones are released or the function of the immune system. However, you can modify your breathing, and this modification sends a signal to the brain and impacts the autonomic nervous system. Slowing your rate of breathing quiets the sympathetic and accentuates the parasympathetic, which means that your mind is quieted, muscles become more relaxed, learning becomes easier and sleep is more restful.

"Coherent breathing" is the term applied to slowing your breathing to about five breaths per minute, which in turn amplifies the parasympathetic system. You calm down, and more importantly, your multiple organs regulated by the autonomic system calm as well.

The process is simple yet can be difficult at first. The idea is to breathe deeply five times per minute by counting slowing to yourself as you breathe — count five in and five out. This can be difficult, especially at first, since it feels unnatural. There are guides that can help. One is called *Respire* found on Amazon Music for free. There are others. This one gives you three choices: listen to a person count for you, listen as a clock and bell tick off the breaths, or listen to two bells that start inspiration and start expiration. Find the option that is most suitable for you.

Give it a try and work your way up to twenty minutes each day. You will notice the difference shortly.

CHAPTER 12: THE MICROBIOME – YOUR NEW BEST FRIEND

"It's not in the stars to find our destiny but in ourselves." - Shakespeare

Let us take a side excursion through your gut to understand the intestinal microbiota (or its gene pool, called the "microbiome," which we will use interchangeably). Its health is critical to your health, and we will refer back to it intermittently in the chapters to follow. Here is a brief microbiota primer.

The human body has multiple "microbiotas," including the major one in the colon (large intestine) plus ones in the mouth, nose, sinuses, vagina and skin. We will focus on the gastrointestinal (GI) microbiome.

Think of your microbiome in the GI tract as an "organ" like your pancreas or gallbladder. It is incredibly important to good health. It takes the fiber your intestines cannot digest and extracts energy for itself and yourself. It produces a variety of critical "postbiotics," such as the short-chain fatty acids called butyrate and acetate, as well as amino acids and vitamins. Your microbiota has major impacts on your metabolism, the maintenance of the intestinal lining and mucosa, inflammation, and the immune system.[18] You want to keep your microbiome healthy so it can help you stay healthy.

An altered microbiome can predispose you to many illnesses, most of them being the complex chronic diseases that impact us as we age, such as type 2 diabetes mellitus, colon cancer, heart disease, Alzheimer's and Parkinson's disease, and non-alcoholic cirrhosis of the liver. It is also intimately involved with obesity, which you have learned is itself a predisposing illness to many other serious maladies.

Damage to the microbiome can occur due to antibiotics, various medications and what you eat. Antibiotics may suppress important bacteria but allow other less desirable bacteria to survive and multiply. Multiple courses of antibiotics over many years can have a devastating effect. It can take years for the microbiome to return to normal, if ever.

A healthy microbiota has immense biodiversity and substantial variation from location to location, even based on the time of day related to the circadian cycle. It also changes due to a variety of external factors that might reach the gut, such as toxins. The microbiota, given its immense size and varied genetics, should be thought of as a second genome with a huge production of messenger RNA that can impact the body's cells for either good or harm. Dysbiosis, or an abnormal alteration of the microbiota, is unhealthy and produces damaging compounds, hinders vitamins and limits the production of healthy compounds such as butyrate, propionate and acetate. Butyrate is an energy source for the intestinal lining cells, is an anti-inflammatory compound, and if it could be patented, would be sold as a "wonder drug." Propionate and acetate are used as energy sources for the heart and the brain. Dysbiosis leads to local inflammation in the gut, can progress to systemic inflammation, can cause "leaky gut" (increased intestinal permeability) and can accentuate chronic inflammation elsewhere in the body. There are many diseases associated with an alteration of the microbiota, including inflammatory bowel diseases, autoimmune diseases, diabetes, obesity, heart diseases, anxiety, depression and many more.

The gut microbiome even has an impact on cancer immunotherapy. New immunomodulating agents called checkpoint inhibitors (which can prevent our helper T cells from recognizing and killing cancer cells) are more effective if the microbiota is healthy. Antibiotics used either before or during treatment reduces efficacy. A specific bacterium called *Akkermansia muciniphila* causes the release of the cytokine IL-2, which in turn seems to "energize" the immune cells. If these bacteria are fed to mice, they respond better to the checkpoint inhibitors. Human studies are underway. Some investigators believe that the absence of antibiotics before treatment could improve response to the drugs by as much as 25-40 percent. If antibiotics are medically required, then perhaps the use of a fecal transplant could rapidly correct the microbiome before treatment.

Maintaining a well-diversified healthy microbiome comes from eating a diet that is well-diversified, especially vegetables that are high in fiber yet low in sugar, and low in foods that are digested rapidly into sugars such as the refined white flour found in most processed foods. These sugars feed the "bad guys" while a limited amount of fiber starves the "good guys." A highly diversified diet with many different vegetables, including different colors and dark leafy greens, and appropriate amounts of fruits, good proteins, and fats with limited refined grains and minimal added sugars will maintain a healthy diverse microbiome.

It is important for the microbiome to be well fed when we are infants and children, as this is when microbial diversity is developed for life. Aberrations can carry forward for years to come. An abnormal microbiome early in life can predispose to multiple allergies, immune abnormalities, and various metabolic diseases as an adult.

Older individuals, especially those in nursing homes, often have microbiomes with markedly reduced diversity. This is associated with frailty and chronic inflammation but cause and effect are unclear. However, it is clear that a monotonous diet, as found in a nursing home and probably in many elders' lives, contributes to reduced microbiome bacterial diversity.

The microbiome of an obese individual is different from others, too, especially with an overabundance of *Firmicutes*. These bacteria have the ability to extract more calories from residual food than those found in higher concentrations in people with a lean physique. As a result, the obese person absorbs more calories from the same food than a thin person. However, if the obese person commits to a long-term change in diet, the microbiota will slowly change back to normal. A recent study found that after a year of following the Mediterranean diet, changes seemed protective of diabetes type 2 due to an increase in certain bacteria such as *Roseburia* and *F prausnitzii*.[19]

Overweight humans often undergo the "yo-yo" effect and lose weight only to have a relapse or recurrence of weight gain a short time later. Obesity leads to a substantial variation in the microbiome composition, and this does not change readily when weight is lost. The microbiome of the obese person degrades dietary flavonoids, which in turn leads to less metabolic activity in fat tissues with lessened energy utilization. If the microbiota can be altered back to "normal," then the flavonoid degradation is also reversed toward normal, and the tendency toward rapid weight regain is reversed.

An interesting recent observation of the microbiome is that it has a circadian regulation.[20] The microbiome actually undergoes variations each day over the course of the circadian rhythm, including variations in the quantities of microbes in different parts of the intestine, different production of metabolites and changes in bacterial access to the systemic circulation. Jet lag, for example, disrupts the normal rhythm and predisposes to glucose intolerance and obesity.

Normally, bacteria or bacterial products cannot cross from the intestines to the bloodstream. However, it is well recognized that both diabetic and obese individuals are susceptible to certain bacteria crossing from the intestines into the systemic bloodstream. Mouse studies have now demonstrated that diabetic animals have a disruption to the normally tight junctions between the intestinal cells that create a barrier to bacteria entering the systemic blood circulation. This appears to be directly related to chronic high levels of blood sugar. In this case, the normally beneficial microbiome becomes a producer of systemic inflammation throughout the body. This finding holds true in humans, and the authors suggest that controlling blood glucose may be key to preventing bacterial contamination of the systemic circulation.[21]

The microbiota also has an impact on the health of the heart and the blood vessels. For example, a study of 893 individuals found that certain families of bacteria had a positive or a negative impact.[22]

When fecal materials were obtained from either healthy or hypertensive individuals and transplanted into germ-free mice, the mice transplanted with the hypertensives' feces developed high blood pressure. There is also evidence that the metabolism created by the microbiota may contribute, in specific individuals, to insulin resistance.[23] Another fascinating observation is that a reduced level of the butyrate-producing bacteria *Ruminococcaceae* correlated with arterial vessel stiffness.[24]

These and other studies are strong reasons to use your diet to improve the diversity of the microbiota since it may prevent some types of heart disease, high blood pressure, obesity, insulin resistance and diabetes. Of course, these are association studies and thus do not necessarily define cause and effect, but they certainly suggest the need for further investigation. In the meantime, it seems logical to use diet, exercise, stress reduction and enhanced sleep to improve the microbiota as much as possible. It also offers the tantalizing potential of fecal transplantation as a means of preventing or treating many diseases.

We will deal with prebiotics and probiotics in the next chapter, but for a moment, let us discuss postbiotics. Postbiotics are those compounds that the microbiota produce via fermentation of your dietary intake and have a biologic activity — positive or negative — on your body.[1,10,12] Foods with probiotics like yogurt create health benefits by fermenting foods and producing natural byproducts. Your microbiota also ferments food products, especially fibrous foods, and produces many valuable compounds. Both prebiotic foods, which the gut bacteria ferment into "postbiotics," and probiotic foods with postbiotics lead to improved immune function, improved infection resistance and protection from a variety of chronic illnesses, including those that cause most of the disabilities and deaths in modern society.

Among the postbiotics created by the microbiota are short-chain fatty acids (SCFAs), various enzymes, proteins, polysaccharides, and vitamins. Short-chain fatty acids such as butyrate and acetate offer energy to intestinal cells and other internal organs, are strong antioxidants and are anti-inflammatory.

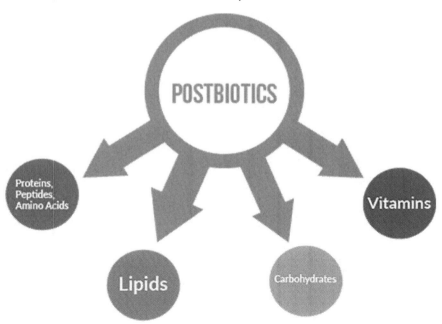

To summarize, although there is still much to be learned about the human microbiota, it is absolutely critical for health.

We will turn next to fiber and its importance in our diet, along with a general discussion of prebiotics and probiotics.

* * *

Ongoing anger is a strong form of persistent stress. Consider forgiveness. It is highly stressful to carry a grudge. Maybe you can resolve the underlying issue with the other person with some open discussion, either together or with a counselor. If that is not practical, look for ways to "just let it go."

The Lord's Prayer includes "forgive us our debts as we forgive our debtors." In other words, the petitioner is not only asking for forgivingness for his or her transgressions but is also committing to forgiving others who may have caused harm.

> *Jennifer was frustrated and angry that her long-time boyfriend had ended their relationship. She was hurt and not sure how to handle it. She had put many years into this relationship and to see it suddenly disappear was stressful, to say the least. Of course, she wondered if it was her fault, but mostly, she blamed him for the breakup. She got back together with Ellen to seek her thoughts. Ellen was polite but direct, saying that she and some of their friends never thought much of the boyfriend but felt it was not appropriate to say so — after all, it was Jenifer's relationship, not theirs. More importantly, she added, if he didn't want to continue the relationship, then it was best to have it end now and not later. Time to move on. And she added, "I know you are angry, but it will only hold you down and hold you back. Don't have persistent anger. Remember the good times you had but then let him go from your life. Easier said than done, but if you do not, that will only harm you, not him. Forgive and move on." Jennifer knew deep down that Ellen was right yet again, but she needed to think this through. But over the next few days, she came to accept the inevitability of the split*

and decided in a flash moment that she would release his hold on her. Once she forgave him by simply letting go of the anger, she felt much better.

CHAPTER 13: PREBIOTICS AND PROBIOTICS AND THE PERFECT POOP

"Everybody looks at their poop." - Oprah Winfrey

Fiber is the non-digestible part of your food. Mostly, it comes from plants such as dark leafy greens, veggies and fruit. Fatty foods, meat and fish have little fiber.

Since most Americans (and everyone else who follows the typical "Western" diet) substantially under-consume vegetables and fruits, most under-consume fiber as well. Nine servings of fruits and veggies will give you enough. It sounds like a lot of veggies, but prior to the overabundance of processed foods high in sugar and white flour, our diet was much higher in fiber and we were healthier because of it.

Prebiotics

Prebiotics are foods that feed your microbiota. Recall that those bacteria love fiber, so prebiotic foods include those with soluble and insoluble fiber in high concentration, such as most vegetables, dark leafy greens, legumes, and fruit. Some specific foods with high levels of prebiotics include flax meal, chicory root, dandelion greens, Jerusalem artichoke, garlic, onions, leeks, asparagus, bananas, barley, oats, apples, wheat bran, seaweed, and cocoa.

Prebiotics can assist the absorption of some minerals such as calcium. By enhancing healthy bacteria, they reduce adverse bacteria in the intestine. But consider that prebiotics are fermented by the bacteria, meaning that if you introduce a large amount at once, you may have bloating. It's better to increase quantity over time.

Today, a remarkable percentage of preschoolers have been found to be constipated. It is an emerging public health problem, and to a large degree, it is related to having too little fiber in the diet.[25] They simply do not eat enough fiber. Lack of fiber in adults is tied to hiatal hernias, reflux esophagitis, diverticular disease, hemorrhoids, and varicose veins. Why? These medical problems all are related to straining with defecation, which increases the intra-abdominal pressure that causes these pressure-induced medical maladies. Increased intra-abdominal pressure is also common among individuals who are overweight or obese, which equates to two-thirds of Americans.

Fiber increases stool size, holds fluid, and makes it easier to pass a bowel movement. Adequate fiber in the diet has been associated with a decreased risk of colon cancer and inflammatory bowel disease. A diet high in fiber lowers circulating estrogen, which could be one of the reasons that women who eat abundant fiber have fewer cases of breast cancer. Men and women who consume a high fiber diet have fewer strokes and a lower rate of heart disease. Soluble fiber reduces LDL cholesterol (the bad kind) by nearly 20 percent, so that may be part of the reason why strokes and heart disease are lower.

Fiber provides more than bulk — it also feeds your colon's good bacteria (see prior chapter). If you feed your bacteria well with good fiber, they produce valuable chemicals that preserve your health. These compounds have anti-inflammatory, anti-cancer, anti-obesity, and blood sugar control effects.

The good bacteria in your gut signal to your immune system, in part, with butyrate. This short-chain fatty acid (more on this later) suppresses the inflammatory reaction. Butyrate calms the immune system, saying in effect, "all's well, you've got the good guys (good bacteria) on board," and ultimately renders the intestinal immune system hypo-responsive to the beneficial bacteria. However, if you do not have enough of this short-chain fatty acid, your immune system becomes activated and chaos ensues.

The total surface area of your gut, if it were to be splayed out, is the surface area of a tennis court at 3,000 square feet! Further, the lining of this large area is only a single cell layer thick. This single layer of enterocytes (the name for the lining cells) separates you from the outside world. This is an interesting concept — the long tube we call the gut is actually "outside," and the gut lining is like your skin. It protects you from chemicals and products entering the body that should not. Those lining cells are replaced with new ones every three to five days. The primary fuel that keeps this single cell layer alive, reproducing, and healthy is butyrate.

You consume some butyrate in your food, but most is produced by the good bacteria in your colon from the fiber you eat. This is a symbiotic relationship that is critical for your good health. You feed your good bacteria well, and in turn, the bacteria make good products to keep you healthy, including anti-inflammatory and immune-modulating chemicals. If you eat junk such as sugar and white flour-based foods, the "bad bacteria" in your gut flourish and produce unhealthy substances that are carcinogenic, inflammatory, and unhealthy for your immune system. Combined, this helps to explain why fiber is anti-inflammatory. So, feed the good bacteria in your gut so they can feed you right back.

When your good bacteria are wiped out by illness, antibiotics, or a particularly poor diet (with predominantly high glycemic index carbohydrates), the bad bacteria take over and start to thrive in your small intestine. Normally, the small (upper) intestine has relatively few bacteria living in it, but antibiotics and the wrong diet can encourage their growth there. This is known as small intestinal bacterial overgrowth, or SIBO, which is being found more frequently because of the Western diet and antibiotic use. Chronic inflammation and increased gut permeability, or "leaky gut," develop alongside SIBO. As a result, bacterial products and parts of the cell wall, which are not supposed to gain entrance to your bloodstream, can enter your circulation, travel to anywhere in the body and cause low grade inflammation in the heart's arteries (with coronary artery disease), joints (with arthritis) or in the brain (with Alzheimer's). Chronic low-grade inflammation is the bedrock for almost all of the chronic illnesses that plague people in their later years. Much of this chronic persistent inflammation can be traced to an altered microbiome. It follows that maintaining a healthy microbiome and avoiding SIBO can go a long way in maintaining good health.

The Flax's of Flax

Some of the earliest cultivated plants were flax. It was known in Babylon at least 5,000 years ago. The Latin name for flax is *Linum usitatissimum,* which translates as "most useful." Apparently, Hippocrates recommended it to his patients with GI issues. The 8th century Holy Roman Emperor, Charlemagne, instructed his subjects to eat flax seeds for their presumed health benefits.

Today, it is appreciated that flax seed and flax meal have multiple health benefits. They can reduce blood pressure, modestly reduce fasting blood sugar, improve lipid composition in the bloodstream and reduce HbA1c levels in those with type 2 diabetes. They may also reduce the risk of breast cancer, decrease menstrual-related breast pain (cyclical mastalgia), help with benign prostatic hypertrophy (BPH or enlarged prostate) and prevent prostate cancer.[2] Plus, flax contains both soluble and insoluble fiber, which is valuable as "food" for your microbiome.

Flax seeds have at least three principal ingredients that offer health benefits: fiber, omega-3 fatty acids, and lignans. To obtain the most

From the Dean Ornish article, see Bibliography, reference #2 benefit, flax meal is better than flax seed, since the seeds are difficult for your body to digest. Flax meal allows access to the nutrients by both your microbiota and your intestinal absorption processes. Some data suggest that flax meal is best uncooked, and you can add it to your food at the end of cooking.

Flax seed contains the long-chain omega-3 fatty acid alpha-linolenic acid (ALA), which is also a precursor to the omega-3 fatty acids DHA (docosahexaenoic acid) and EPA (eicosapentaenoic acid). These are anti-inflammatory substances and critical for brain development, maintenance, and function. Unfortunately, humans cannot rapidly convert ALA to DHA or EPA, so less than 4 percent of the ALA in flax is metabolized to those two omega-3 fatty acids.[26] You must, therefore, get your DHA and EPA from a fish or algal supplement.

ALA itself is valuable to your health. It appears to protect against cardiac and vascular diseases and reduce cholesterol levels and chronic inflammation. It also appears that ALA levels correlate with a lower risk of breast cancer, though there is controversy as to whether ALA may increase or decrease the risk of prostate cancer. Another benefit may be a reduction in the resorption of bone minerals. ALA is an essential fatty acid and cannot be made de novo by the human cell — we have to get it from our food.

Lignans are part of the structure of plant cell walls. The lignans in food, called phytoestrogens, are converted by intestinal bacteria into enterolactone, which can be absorbed into the circulation where it has weak estrogen activity. It is believed that this activity is the basis for the observation that lignans help to prevent cancer, heart disease and other ailments and diseases. Flax contains 75 to 800 times more lignans than any other plant food. Lignans have anti-cancer properties along with estrogen and antioxidant effects. For more information, refer to the two videos in these references that relate flax to breast cancer[27] and to prostate cancer.[28]

If you are eating well, staying well hydrated and getting a reasonable amount of fiber, particularly from veggies, fruits, flax, beans and nuts, chances are your bowel habit is good.

What is a normal bowel movement? It is the rule of three: from three times per day to three times per week. You are what you eat and drink. Digested and undigested liquid food (known as chyme) leaves the stomach and works its way through the long absorptive tunnel of the small bowel. Until it reaches your large intestine, it remains a liquid. The small bowel is where the food is further digested into its base elements such as sugars, fatty acids, and amino acids. Once in that form, they can be absorbed into the bloodstream and used by the body's cells.

The main function of the large intestine is to be a reservoir of your microbiome, hopefully, a healthy microbiome. The large bowel (colon) is a highly bioactive site that holds two to three pounds of bacteria! The indigestible food left after the small bowel does its work enters the colon and provides nutrients to those trillions of bacteria that use the leftover food to make good or bad compounds, which benefit or damage your health. If you eat poorly, the bacteria are being fed poorly, and they make chemicals that can have mutagenic effects (damage your DNA), carcinogenic effects (predispose to cancer), and inflammatory effects (damage any part of the body). Conversely, if you eat appropriately, those bacteria will reward you with compounds that improve your immunity, protect and energize the lining cells of the colon and more. It is all about what you eat!

In addition, the large intestine absorbs water from what remains, just the right amount so you will have a perfect movement. This should be a somewhat firm, smooth, light brown cylinder that is easy to pass without straining and plops into the toilet. If perfect, you may not even need to wipe! Often stool has some undigested material, but 60 percent of the dry weight of poop is dead bacteria. Your stool size and consistency say a lot about your health.

Medically, we use the Bristol stool scale to grade poop. The perfect poop is a 3 to 4. Take a look!

Bristol Stool Chart

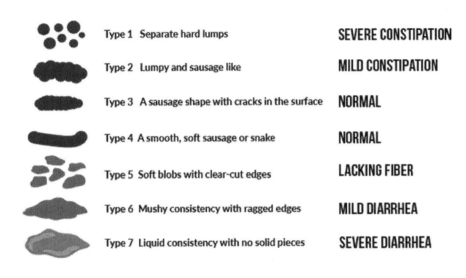

Type 1	Separate hard lumps	SEVERE CONSTIPATION
Type 2	Lumpy and sausage like	MILD CONSTIPATION
Type 3	A sausage shape with cracks in the surface	NORMAL
Type 4	A smooth, soft sausage or snake	NORMAL
Type 5	Soft blobs with clear-cut edges	LACKING FIBER
Type 6	Mushy consistency with ragged edges	MILD DIARRHEA
Type 7	Liquid consistency with no solid pieces	SEVERE DIARRHEA

You may have noticed that many older people eat prunes to aid bowel movements. Is it just an old wives' tale or is there something to it? Prunes (dried plums) have a modest amount of both soluble and insoluble fiber in them, so they are not on the list of high-fiber foods. So, what makes them useful? Probably it is the sorbitol and the phenolics in them. Sorbitol is a sugar alcohol that is not digested in the small intestine but creates an osmotic pull to bring in added water. This means that when the remaining nondigested food reaches the colon, it is more liquid, which may be the explanation for their effectiveness with constipation. Four or five prunes contain about six grams of sorbitol, and prune juice has about 15 grams in an eight-ounce glass but is missing the insoluble fiber. In one study, twenty grams produced diarrhea in half of normal subjects, so be careful with how many you eat. Sorbitol in the colon is partially fermented by the microbiota and may cause gas and bloating. And do not forget that prunes are high in fructose.

Probiotics

Probiotics are living microorganisms, mostly bacteria, which, upon ingestion in adequate numbers, exert health effects beyond basic nutrition. The concept of probiotics was first reported by Nobel Prize-winning physiologist Elie Metchnikoff, PhD, in 1907. Metchnikoff is generally credited with first recognizing that certain blood cells called macrophages ingest and destroy bacteria and is thought of as the father of cellular immunity. Among his many works, Metchnikoff postulated that consumption of fermented milk products such as yogurt is responsible for the longevity of certain ethnic groups. He also suggested that these products manipulate the intestinal microflora to maintain the normal balance between pathogenic (bad or disease-causing) and nonpathogenic (healthy) bacteria.

Most foods with natural probiotic bacteria contain a variety of strains of lactobacilli and bifidobacteria. Foods that naturally contain probiotics include yogurt (fermented milk), kefir (also fermented milk), buttermilk, sauerkraut, kimchi (the Korean style of sauerkraut), sour pickles (the kind not made from vinegar but from salt and water brine), brine-cured olives, kombucha (a type of fermented tea), miso (based on fermented soybeans), tempeh (also based on fermented soybeans), natto (another Japanese dish from fermented soybeans), sourdough bread (the starter), some soft cheeses like Gouda and raw cheeses from goat's milk, sheep's milk or A2 cow's milk and possibly apple cider vinegar. Dark cholate is sometimes touted as a probiotic because the cacao beans are fermented with probiotic bacteria, but they are almost always killed when the chocolate is heated in the next stage of the processing. According to some, the foods with the most probiotic potential are sauerkraut, kimchi and pickles, followed by kefir, yogurt, buttermilk, and raw cheese. Next is tempeh, natto and kombucha, followed by cottage cheese (although almost all commercially available cottage cheese has been pasteurized), miso (effective only if added to the soup at the last minute so as not to boil away the beneficial microbes), and sourdough (since most of the probiotic organisms are killed by the baking of the bread).

If you are looking to purchase food with probiotics, be sure to notice if the label says "live active cultures." Many products are fermented but then the probiotic bacteria are destroyed before packaging. Yogurt that has added fruits, sugars or vanilla is almost always bacteria free. Sauerkraut in cans is rendered sterile, as are most jarred pickles.

Probiotic bacteria can be packaged in capsule form. Grocery stores, health food stores and pharmacies often have many varieties. Which one to buy and at what dose is unclear, although some combination of various lactobacilli and bifidobacteria are likely good choices. In the future, specific recommendations will be based on each person's situation, but for now, it is best to select from reputable manufacturers. How to choose? Go to a store with a knowledgeable individual who can guide you, hopefully in a nonbiased manner. Do be wary of internet hype, which is abundant.

Probiotic-rich foods or capsules containing probiotic bacteria must pass through the stomach's acid milieu, where many are destroyed. Certain bacteria, including the lactobacilli and bifidobacteria, survive the stomach's acid, as do some of the bacteria in yogurt and other natural probiotics foods. Compared to the 100 trillion bacteria in the gut, the numbers in probiotic foods or capsules are dwarfed. Still, they do have an impact.

Probiotic organisms that survive the stomach and upper small intestine can impact the microbiota composition, improve your immune system and inactivate mutagenic and carcinogenic substances. Probiotics have been shown to be effective in the treatment of several forms of diarrhea, including rotaviral and other forms of diarrhea in children, antibiotic-associated diarrhea in children and travelers' diarrhea. Some individuals develop a very severe form of relapsing *Clostridium difficile* ("C. diff") diarrhea, usually as a result of intensive antibiotic use. This has been exceptionally difficult to control, but recently, probiotic enemas or fecal "transplants" by enema have brought lasting resolution. These placebo-controlled studies suggest that modulating the colonic bacteria can have important, valuable implications.

Probiotic capsules may be valuable, but remember, your diet affects your intestinal bacteria composition. Sugar, high fructose corn syrup, refined grains (white flour), packaged and processed foods (often made with sugars and flour) and meat and poultry that were fed antibiotics can each negatively impact your microbiome.

What does all this mean? Fix your diet first! Then consider added measures to improve the microbiota/microbiome. Load up on prebiotic foods to feed the good bacteria in your gut. Cut back on sugar and white flour-based foods to starve the "bad guys." Then add in probiotic foods, and finally, if your physician recommends it, take probiotic capsules. But to repeat, eat a healthy diet along the lines of what we recommend in this book, and be sure it is packed with prebiotic and probiotic foods.

* * *

You probably get a fasting blood sugar test done at your annual exam with your primary care physician. A new study from researchers at Stanford University put continuous glucose monitors on otherwise healthy people and found that many have intermittent spikes in their blood sugar — which neither they nor their doctor expected. Although it was not measured, we can assume each spike was followed by an insulin spike. These two events are risk factors for coronary artery disease and other diseases and can lead to insulin resistance. In the study, each person responded with sugar spikes from different carbohydrate foods, but one food that caused spikes in 80 percent of people was a breakfast of corn flakes and milk. Michael Snyder, PhD, the lead investigator of the study, suggested that "understanding the microbiome and manipulating it is going to be a big part of this, and that's where our research is headed next."[29] Snyder said that most people might benefit from a continuous glucose monitoring test annually.

* * *

Strengthening Your Transverse Abdominus Muscle

Let us take a step back for a moment and give you a reminder of the importance of a strong transverse abdominus muscle. It gives structure and support to your belly, improves your posture, and helps you sit up straight. Here is a different video that shows another method to strengthen your TA. The one in the earlier chapter can be done multiple times each day, and this one is good perhaps twice per day. It has the advantage of building up most of your core muscles, and the other one is quick and easy no matter where you are, such as the supermarket checkout lane. Use them both.

https://www.youtube.com/watch?v=yZteoscSIpk

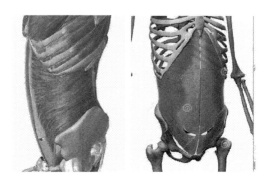

CHAPTER 14: SLEEP

"Sleep is the best meditation." - Dalai Lama

Jennifer usually slept soundly each night. She lived in an apartment where her neighbors were rarely noisy, and her shades and curtains meant the bedroom was dark except for her cell phone and alarm. Although she rarely had to take work home at night, she did always check her emails before bed and then looked at Facebook. She had a TV on the wall opposite her bed where she usually watched the 11 p.m. news and the start of the Late Show so she would drift off to sleep about 12:15 or so. Her digital alarm on her bedside table was set for 6:30 a.m. Most of her work colleagues were proud of the fact that they could get by easily on about five-and-a-half to six hours of sleep.

When our immune system is working optimally, it defends us against infections, cancer, and inflammation. It also allows us to age gracefully instead of decaying and deteriorating. Critical to the immune system are the four pillars of health: good nutrition, regular exercise, stress management and restorative sleep. Let us now turn to sleep.

We spend about a third of our lives sleeping (about twenty-six years). Sleep repairs and rejuvenates our bodies. For most adults, seven to eight hours of sleep per night seems to be the correct amount. Sleep deprivation can cause a number of chronic conditions. It can weaken your immune system, accelerate tumor growth, and contribute to a pre-diabetic state that makes you feel hungry. Sleep deprivation can impair memory and performance on physical and mental tasks, enhance anxiety and depression, and accentuate chronic pain. You are dependent upon adequate sleep for your social, emotional, and behavioral skills the next day. In short, sleep is absolutely critical, but most of society does not recognize its importance.

Some people claim they can get by on very limited sleep, say three to four hours. Frankly, they are fooling only themselves. Many careful studies have proven that reaction time, attentiveness, memory recall, and concentration all decline with inadequate sleep.

The sleep cycle is a complex process. Each cycle of deep sleep (known as NREM) lasts about an hour or so and is followed by rapid eye movement (REM) sleep that lasts 15-20 minutes for a total cycle of about ninety minutes. Then, there is a brief period of being nearly awake, followed by another deep NREM sleep period and a REM period. As the night progresses, the REM sleep time increases so the later cycles might be 110-120 minutes long. Healthy sleep usually consists of five to six cycles per night.

NREM sleep has four stages. Each phase is a deeper sleep:

- Stage I sleep is non-restorative. You may know it as dozing as you can be easily awakened. Although your muscle tone relaxes, you may have some muscle "jerk."

- Stage II is deeper and you cannot be aroused as easily. Your body temperature and heart rate begin to decline, and your eyes become motionless. Stage II sleep is known as spindle sleep because of its distinctive appearance of slow brain waves with intermittent spikes called spindles on an electroencephalogram (EEG). Stage II sleep is important for memory refreshment and consolidation. Think of writing a letter on a computer. When finished, you must click on "save as" and find a folder and perhaps a subfolder that you can access easily and logically. Your brain is doing the same thing in this stage of sleep. The hippocampus holds the temporary memories of the day just as the RAM of the computer. During sleep, it selects the important memories and moves them into the cortex (the hard drive) in a location where they can be found. The more sleep spindles during Stage II sleep, the better you can learn the next day. Most of the sleep spindles come in the later cycles of the night, so if you lose the last one or two cycles with an early wakeup, you lose valuable learning effectiveness the next day. Stage II is also important for consolidating skill or automatic activities such as walking, piano playing, surgical prowess, and even eating. This also occurs mostly in the later cycles of the sleep pattern and emphasizes the importance of getting enough cycles per night.

- Stage III and IV sleep are known as deep sleep or slow wave sleep (SWS). This is when the body truly has restoration. The EEG is distinctive for slow waves. It is during this time that your catecholamines levels (epinephrine and norepinephrine) and cortisol levels fall. Rational thinking is one of the last parts of the brain to fully develop, and sleep is critical to its occurrence. Poor quality deep sleep leads to physical and cognitive problems. Deep sleep is when "synaptic pruning" takes place and the brain embarks on the process of cleaning up unwanted or unneeded connections. This is very important for adolescents to reach maturity, and until these excess synapses are pruned, teens tend to take greater risks and make poorer decisions.

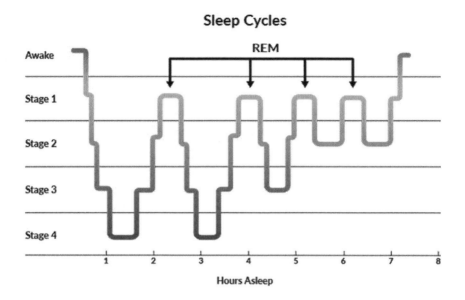

Sleep Cycles

Awake · REM · Stage 1 · Stage 2 · Stage 3 · Stage 4

Hours Asleep

In REM (rapid eye movement) sleep, you can be more easily awakened, yet your body is largely paralyzed except for the movement of your eyes and muscular movement related to breathing. REM sleep is also called dream sleep, and the EEG is very similar to the EEG of being awake. REM sleep is critical for your emotional health. This is when recent emotionally-charged memories are tempered. The memory persists, but the negative connotations of the memory are diminished. Think of the phrase "time heals all wounds."

REM sleep is when creativity can occur. During normal wakefulness, your brain can only think in linear terms, but in REM sleep, it can and does pull together various thoughts and memories, both recent and long past, from all parts of the brain. It integrates them and allows you to "see" differently. Without good REM sleep, it is unusual to be creative the next day.

The first of these cycles lasts about 90 minutes, and the remainder may consume 100 to 120 minutes, with the REM sleep stage lengthening with each cycle. You need about five cycles (7 ½ to 8 ½ hours) to be refreshed the following day. It is simply not correct that you can set your alarm, get up early and "skip" that last cycle without significant harm to your physiology.

Children and adolescents need longer total sleep time. Adolescents are hampered because they are expected to get up early to catch the school bus, but their circadian rhythm is different than adults. They need a longer total sleep time (about 9-9 ½ hours) and they tend to go to sleep later than adults, but their school schedule forces them to awaken at least an hour or so earlier than adults. They are not necessarily lazy, just following their natural rhythms. If they lose that last cycle of sleep, they will tend to be less able to learn and less able to handle emotional situations. School systems in Seattle ran an experiment by pushing high school start times about an hour later. The result? Students got an average of 34 more minutes of sleep, better attendance, and better grades.[30]

Older individuals also have some disadvantages related to sleep. After the first cycle, the following cycles do not drop into as deep a sleep. Between cycles, they tend to awaken and head for the bathroom to urinate, so their sleep is not efficient, and they need more time in bed to get the required five or more cycles of sleep. Poor sleep is an important contributor to cognitive decline, along with some of the age prevalent chronic diseases such as type 2 diabetes, cardiovascular disease, cancer, and Alzheimer's disease.

When your body's natural rhythms are disrupted, you produce less melatonin. Melatonin is a hormone released by the pineal gland and is a powerful antioxidant. This means that melatonin suppresses free radical formation. Free radicals are generated by oxidation and can be harmful to your body. A healthy source of melatonin is dried tart cherries. They can be helpful, especially when changing time zones. Try a handful thirty to forty-five minutes before retiring for the night. Light, including blue light from your phone, tablet, TV, and computer, inhibits the release of melatonin from your pineal gland. Sleep in the dark!

Growth hormone levels rise with deep sleep. Sleep deprivation prematurely ages you by interfering with your growth hormone secretion. Studies have shown that people with chronic insomnia have triple the risk of dying from any cause.

Obstructive sleep apnea is a condition that often affects overweight and obese people. In this condition, the airway collapses during inhalation and affects breathing. This causes an inability to breathe (apnea) and carbon dioxide (CO_2) increases in the blood and triggers the brain to wake up momentarily. This can cause frequent short pulses of adrenaline hormones, which disrupt your ability to achieve deep sleep. This can affect your immune system, memory, and physical performance. In addition, it drives up ghrelin levels and leads to overeating. This typically causes cravings for starchy and sweet food. Eating these types of foods elevates your serotonin, dopamine, insulin, and leptin levels. This promotes weight gain and causes a worsening of sleep apnea.

Mono-phasic Sleep Versus Polyphasic Sleep

Most mammals are polyphasic sleepers, meaning they sleep for short periods throughout the day. Humans, however, are part of the minority that are largely mono-phasic sleepers. Our days are divided into two distinct periods: one for sleep and one for wakefulness.

Are we really monophasic? Over the last 300-400 years, there has been a shift, which began when timepieces were invented and we no longer used the sun and the sundial to keep time. Young children and elderly persons typically nap. In modern times, napping is unusual, but it can be very restorative. So maybe we really are polyphasic sleepers. Further, lack of sleep or poor sleep continuity contributes to our daytime tired state. Among other things, daytime fatigue that is caused by sleep deprivation (less than six hours per night) has been shown to increase insulin levels. This, of course, makes it more difficult to lose weight. Fatigue also causes ghrelin secretion that causes cravings for carbohydrates.

Napping

We are a sleep-deprived nation, and it may be that our busy lifestyles keep us from napping. Although napping will not necessarily make up for inadequate or poor-quality nighttime sleep, a short nap of twenty to thirty minutes can improve mood, alertness, and performance. Naps can also reduce mistakes and accidents due to sleep deprivation and provide an easy way to get some relaxation and rejuvenation.

Driving while sleepy (and with heavy eyes) is extremely dangerous. Still, many drivers press on when they feel drowsy in spite of the risks, putting themselves and others in harm's way. Heavy eyes are a warning and an alert that microsleeps might happen, which can last for less than a second or a bit more. But while you are in that state, just like when you are in deep sleep, the connection between the brain's motor cortex and the muscles are turned off. You are no longer in control of your car. Imagine that in two seconds you can be driving in the opposing lane or have slipped off the side of the road into a ditch — all in that limited time when you were "asleep." We think of drunk driving as especially dangerous, and of course, it is. But microsleeps lead to about six times more fatal accidents. The real problem is that most individuals do not realize how dangerous these microsleeps can be. Truckers are especially prone to them because they tend to drive long hours, and since many are obese, they are prone to sleep apnea. While getting a full night's sleep before driving is ideal, taking a short nap before driving can reduce a person's risk of having a drowsy driving crash. Sleep experts also recommend that if you feel drowsy when driving, you should immediately pull over to a rest area, drink a caffeinated beverage and take a twenty-minute nap.

Naps can leave people with sleep inertia when the nap lasts longer than thirty minutes. Sleep inertia is the feeling of grogginess and disorientation that can come with awakening from a deep sleep, like being awakened by a loud noise at 4 a.m. When this occurs, the body's sleep cycle is interrupted, resulting in diminished functions and extreme grogginess. It can also occur if you sleep too long. While this state usually only lasts for a few minutes to half an hour, it can be detrimental to those who must perform immediately after waking from a nap. If you decide to use a nap to refresh yourself, keep it to about twenty minutes.

Sleep Pressure

Melatonin, produced in the pineal gland of the brain in response to lessened light, sends a message to the body that it is dark and time to sleep. But melatonin itself does not produce sleep — that is the result of adenosine.

During the day, brain cells produce a chemical called adenosine. It is a normal byproduct of energy expenditure. Adenosine attaches to the surface of brain cells and creates a sense of needing to sleep, which is called sleep pressure. As the day progresses and more adenosine is created, the sleep pressure builds up. Once asleep and the brain cells are less active, the adenosine is enzymatically degraded. By the time you wake up after a full night's sleep, the adenosine levels are very low and you do not feel "sleepy." But then the cycle begins again. Caffeine locks onto the same receptors on the brain cells, preventing the newly produced adenosine from attaching. This is the essence of caffeine's effectiveness, although it is also a direct stimulant. Once the caffeine dissipates, usually after five to seven hours or more, the adenosine now attaches, and the sense of sleep pressure recurs. Drinking caffeine-loaded drinks such as coffee, tea, sodas, and energy drinks later in the day can affect your ability to fall asleep because it is still attached to the brain receptors, preventing the normal sleep pressure of adenosine.

Optimizing Your Sleep

Here are some suggestions to enhance your sleep:

- Keep to a regular schedule of retiring and arising. Routine is helpful in achieving good sleep.

- Play some relaxing music before bedtime.

- Avoid violent, horror and other excitatory TV shows before bedtime. Watch humor instead.

- Similarly, do not read books or articles before bedtime that are "downers."

- Strive to obtain about 7.5 to 8 hours of sleep each night.

- Use the bedroom only for sleep, not for watching television, checking Facebook or other tasks.

- Keep the temperature in the bedroom no higher than 70 degrees, and optimal is 65.

- The bedroom should be completely dark and completely quiet. Get good shades for the window. Turn off your digital alarm, computer, smartphone, and iPad — they emit a blue light that impacts your sleep cycle. Use an eye mask if necessary.

- Just before dozing off, think about gratitude.

- Use melatonin an hour before bed, if necessary.

- Do not drink caffeine after noon, and limit fluids for the two hours before bed.

- Allow three hours to elapse between the end of dinner and bedtime.

- In the hours before bedtime, avoid foods that contain tyramine, an amino acid that stimulates the brain to release norepinephrine, activates brain activity and inhibits the start of sleep. Some examples are sausage, salami, bacon, corned beef, pickled herring, smoked fish, pepperoni, overripe fruits and vegetables, and sauerkraut. Other tyramine-containing foods are red wine, many highly aged cheeses, eggplant, and soy sauce. As long as you allow about three hours between supper and bedtime, the effects of these foods will probably be minimal, but everyone is different.

- Do not exercise close to bedtime. It will overstimulate your system with catecholamines.

- Obtain a healthy weight. Yes, this is more difficult than the above, but being overweight has a negative impact on sound sleep and can induce sleep apnea.

* * *

Free Radicals and Oxidation

When you cut into an apple, it soon turns brown, which is oxidation. Obviously, this is a natural process. All molecules have a certain number of electrons. If one is lost, that molecule wants to find one to replace the lost one. The molecule with a missing electron is called a "free radical," and although also perfectly normal, large quantities can disrupt cellular machinery and damage DNA. Free radicals lead to inflammation, which is the root of nearly every chronic disease. What leads to too many free radicals? Smoking, too much alcohol, excess chronic stress, not enough sleep, pollution and many of the commonly-sold processed foods. Of course, other than pollution, these can be controlled to a major extent by adjusting your lifestyle.

The body's normal process of controlling free radicals and oxidation is with antioxidants, which are primarily found in foods or created from those foods. The major antioxidants are vitamins A, C, E, Coenzyme Q and others. Certain minerals are important as well, including selenium, copper, and zinc.

A diet rich in vegetables of various types and colors is your key to reducing oxidation and excess free radical formation and quelling inflammation.

Jennifer began to realize that she was not getting enough sleep. Her late-to-bed and early-to-rise schedule meant she was getting at most six hours of sleep each night. She wondered how much that inadequate sleep was affecting her hunger and her weight, which was something she had never considered in the past. She decided to go to bed earlier with lights out by 11 p.m. but kept her alarm set for 6:30 a.m. She started watching TV only in the living room, turned off her cell phone at bedtime and turned the digital clock so it faced away from her. Facebook and email checks were ended at 7 p.m.

CHAPTER 15: FAT

**"For the first time ever, overweight people outnumber average
people in America. Doesn't that make overweight the average
then? Last month you were fat, now you're average — hey, let's
get a pizza!"** - Jay Leno

Before we get into a discussion about fats, let us pause for a moment
and consider some basic ways to think and act to improve your
overall health.

Yes, you probably want to lose some weight, and yes, you probably
want to reduce your "overfat." But this is not about being cosmetic
so you can fit into a slimmer swimsuit. No, it should be about how
you can have the best possible health today and in the future.

In order to claim success, it is necessary to set goals and define the
measures that indicate success or a "job well done." You might have
noticed that we have not discussed weighing yourself. That is because
the basic message of BOOM is not really about weight but about
adjusting your lifestyle. The measurement that should be most
important to you is this: "How am I doing with these adjustments
and modifications?"

If you are eating a better diet loaded with vegetables, fruits, healthy
oils, fin fish and very limited sugars and flours, then you have made a

valuable shift! If you are taking a daily walk and doing twice weekly resistance exercises, that's terrific. Congratulate yourself! And better yet if you have reduced your carb intake further and are doing the HIIT regularly after a prolonged overnight fast. These are the important measurements. If you can make this shift in your daily living, then your health will improve, you will feel more energetic and life will seem much better. Let the weight take care of itself — it will.

We will discuss some additional modifications to achieve shortly, especially related to stress and sleep.

For now, you are in the process of changing your habits and modifying your lifestyle. This can be difficult, but it is certainly not impossible. Start slow. We have tried to help you by making the BOOM program iterative and adding in a new element each week rather than everything all at once. If you cannot keep up, that is okay. Simply continue at whatever point you are at, and then after a few more sessions, add the next step. Do not feel pressured, but of course, do not assume that you can wait "forever" to move up the ladder. Think in terms of being "additive" rather than "restrictive." For example, instead of concentrating on reducing carbs, think in terms of increasing healthy foods such as dark leafy greens and vegetables. This will allow you to grab the "low hanging fruit," which in turn will increase your confidence. Keep at it! You can do it and the end result will be gratifying.

A Fat Primer

Fats are essential for your health. Dietary fats are mostly triglycerides (about 90 percent of daily fat intake) but also cholesterol (about 10 percent), and a variety of others that combine to make up a small proportion of daily fat intake. You need to consume some of the right kinds of triglycerides every day. They are critical for your brain, which is made up mostly of fats, the membranes of all of your cells, your heart muscle and general cellular integrity. Cholesterol is the building block for many hormones, including estrogen and testosterone.

Fat Composition

Triglycerides are composed of three elements — carbon, oxygen, and hydrogen. That is it, and it is the same as carbohydrates but arranged differently. The type of fat depends on how and how many of these three elements are linked together, so consider a bit of chemistry. Carbon has four bonding points, oxygen has two and hydrogen has one. This means that carbon can hold four hydrogens (CH4 or methane), oxygen can hold two (H2O or water), and carbon can hold two hydrogens and one oxygen. Visualize it here:

H- and H-   =C=   -O-

Note that the two carbons can either hold six hydrogens or they can double bond with each other and hold four hydrogens. The former is termed "saturated" while the latter is called "unsaturated." That is the essence of what makes a fat saturated or unsaturated. Exactly where the double-bonded carbons are located and how many of them exist will determine the type of fatty acid.

H3-C-C-H3   H2-C=C-H2

Fatty acids are long chains of carbons and hydrogens, and at one end is a complex of one carbon with two oxygens and one hydrogen known as a carboxyl group, or an acid, which creates the term "fatty acid."

COOH

Butyric acid has a full complement of hydrogens and is a saturated fatty acid. Oleic has one double-bond between two carbons, thus eliminating two hydrogens and is monounsaturated. Linoleic acid has two positions with double bonds between carbons and is polyunsaturated.

C-C-C-COOH   Butyric Acid (Saturated)

C-C-C-C-C-C-C-C-C=C-C-C-C-C-C-C-C-COOH Oleic acid (Monounsaturated)

C-C-C-C-C-C-C-C-C=C-C-C=C-C-C-C-C-COOH Linoleic Acid (Polyunsaturated)

Saturated fatty acids tend to be straight whereas the double bonds of unsaturated fatty acids allow them to "kink" or bend. The saturated fat in a piece of grain-fed beef or butter is firm when cool whereas the unsaturated fat of a fish is soft and pliable and that of vegetable oils are liquid.

Fats are composed of three fatty acids attached to a glycerol molecule and are termed triglycerides.

3 Fatty Acids + Glycerol

Fat Digestion and Absorption

When you eat a fat (a.k.a. a lipid), it is digested with an enzyme called lipase, beginning with oral lipase, then further digestion in the stomach with emulsification. It continues in the small intestine with intestinal and pancreatic lipase and is aided by bile salts. The lipase breaks the fat into its three constituent fatty acids and glycerol. These can be absorbed by the intestinal lining cells, where they are reformed into triglycerides, packaged in special carriers called chylomicrons, and sent into the lymphatic system and finally into the bloodstream. When they reach cells such as a muscle cell, another form of lipase breaks them down into fatty acids again, which can be absorbed

127

across the capillary membrane into the muscle cell. There they can be used as an energy source.

Fatty Acids as an Energy Source

Like glucose, fatty acids can be used by cells as an energy source. The fatty acids are broken down in the cell's mitochondria into smaller pieces, which in turn can be converted into energy in biologic processes such as muscle contraction. Fats produce nine calories of energy per gram whereas carbohydrates and proteins produce five.

Most fatty acids are too long to pass through the blood-brain barrier and so are of no use to the brain, but medium-chain length fatty acids that make up so-called medium-chain triglycerides can be utilized.

Fatty Acids and Fat Cells

When you eat a high carbohydrate diet of sugar and white flour, any glucose not used by cells for energy immediately is stored in the liver as glycogen. But when the liver's storage capacity is filled, the excess glucose is sent to fat cells where it is converted into and stored as fatty acids and glycerol forming triglycerides. It is interesting to note that most body fat is not the result of eating a diet high in fats but rather eating a diet high in rapidly digested and absorbed carbohydrates.

When your body is low on glucose, or when you have not eaten recently and your blood sugar drops because liver glycogen stores have been depleted, your body starts breaking down fats that have been stored in adipose (fat) cells. Many of these compounds of fat breakdown can be used by cells for energy. Ketones (loosely called "ketone bodies," although they are not "bodies" but organic chemicals) are one of the products of this breakdown of fatty acids into short-chain compounds of three or four carbon lengths. Ketone bodies (Acetoacetate and β-Hydroxy butyrate) are released into the circulation and are then used by cells, including in the brain, muscle, and heart, as an energy source in the absence of glucose.

Types of Triglycerides

There are four different types of fats:

- Saturated fat, which comes from animal products and tropical plants, such coconuts.

- Mono-unsaturated fat, such as olive oil.

- Poly-unsaturated fat, such as omega-3 and omega-6 fatty acids that largely come from plants, especially algae.

- Trans-fats, such as margarine, which are man-made from vegetable oils.

Saturated Fats

Studies over the past sixty years have correlated saturated fats with an increased risk of coronary artery disease and other diseases. The result of these studies became a series of recommendations by the government and voluntary organizations that saturated fats be reduced in the diet. Unfortunately, the recommendations then called for a reduction of all fats and replacement of the lost energy values with carbohydrates such as breads and cereals. This may have been a tragic error. It was only saturated fats that were found to be associated with disease, not all fats. But with increased ingestion of carbohydrates, the obesity epidemic began. Of course, it was not just carbohydrates — obesity came from a huge increase in the consumption of sugar and refined white flour, a shift from three to six meals per day, the lack of eating as a family event, the rise of fast food restaurants and other factors.

It is interesting that coronary heart disease deaths have fallen since the 1950s in America while at the same time weight gain and obesity have advanced rapidly. In countries where saturated fats were reduced and replaced with unsaturated fats (such as Finland) without corresponding increases in carbohydrates, rates of heart disease dropped substantially, and longevity increased by a decade. Of course, there may be other factors involved.

Monounsaturated Fat

The most common example is olive oil, which contains a high percentage of oleic acid, but monounsaturated fats are also present in many other foods such as beef and eggs. Monounsaturated fatty acids are fundamentally healthy and have little or no adverse consequences unless one consumes so much that it affects caloric balance. Olive oil is the oil of choice for salad dressings and low heat cooking.

Polyunsaturated Fats

There are many polyunsaturated fats, but you hear mostly about those that are either omega-6 or omega-3 fatty acids. It is the omega-3 fatty acids found in fin fish like salmon, mackerel, and sardines that are recognized as heart-healthy. The omega-6 fatty acids are found mostly in vegetables. They, too, are important for health but not in the quantities that the average American consumes today.

Omega-3 and Omega-6 Fatty Acids

Your body can produce from glucose all of its required fatty acids except for linoleic acid (LA), an omega-6 fatty acid, and alpha-linolenic acid (ALA), an omega-3 fatty acid. These have to be consumed from the diet and are therefore termed "essential fatty acids."

Consumption of omega-6 fatty acids has increased over the last 70-150 years while the intake of omega-3 fatty acids has decreased. This change parallels the increase in coronary artery disease, although as we have indicated repeatedly, it is important to note that association does not necessarily equate with causation.

Most of what we term "vegetable oils," from rapeseed (canola), soybeans, corn, and sunflower, are polyunsaturated. These oils are extracted with a chemical process. There is controversy about whether the manufacturing process for extracting the oils can damage the fatty acids and make them less healthy. Many would say they are fine, and others would say the opposite.

By contrast, the oils from olives and coconuts can be extracted by pressing without the need for chemical processing.

Trans Fats

Trans fats are man-made usually from liquid vegetable oils. The basic process, developed about 100 years ago, is to bubble hydrogen gas through the oil, which turns it into a semisolid or solid-state and gives it the name of "partially hydrogenated" vegetable oils. By adding the hydrogen, the fatty acids become saturated but in a different configuration called "trans" rather than the natural "cis" configuration of saturated fats, hence the name "trans fats." Good examples are margarine and Crisco. Their advantage is long shelf life, so they are used in many pastries, donuts, cakes and pies that are on the grocery shelf. The concept was that vegetable oils were presumed healthy, and if they could be made into a solid, it would be easy to store, use and preserve for weeks, months or even years. Our mothers and grandmothers used them to make terrific pie crusts that were light and flakey. Hydrogenated oils are also often used for deep fat frying in fast food restaurants.

The end result, however, is that hydrogenated oils are completely unnatural and cause cellular dysfunction. A comprehensive review of studies of trans fats was published in 2006 in the *New England Journal of Medicine*, which showed a strong, reliable connection between trans-fat consumption and coronary artery disease. A brief but excellent review and discussion of these fats can be found in an article from the Harvard School of Public Health.[31]

Trans fats have been proven to be harmful to human health by inciting chronic inflammation, adversely impacting the inner lining of blood vessels, and creating insulin resistance.

Some political jurisdictions such as New York City have banned them. Many fast food restaurants are or have already found substitutes for deep fat production of French fries, fried chicken, and other friend foods. A good rule of thumb is to avoid foods with trans fats, and fortunately, nutrition labels must now indicate their presence.

Cholesterol is an essential building block for many hormones. Although some of the cholesterol circulating in the bloodstream is from the diet, most is created in the liver. Each person has a "set point" like a thermostat for cholesterol. Eat less and the liver makes more; eat more and the liver makes less. This balancing helps to explain why avoiding dietary cholesterol often does not reduce circulating cholesterol (although it is effective for some people). The amount of cholesterol made in the liver depends to a large degree on one's ingestion of certain triglycerides, and of course, one's genetic composition. Consuming trans fats, saturated fat, sugar, and foods that convert quickly to sugar can all increase your LDL ("bad") cholesterol level. Excess weight predisposes to a rise in LDL and a drop in HDL ("good") cholesterol. Exercise leads to the reverse with a drop in LDL and rise in HDL.

* * *

It is important to remember that fats are crucial elements of your diet. They are necessary for brain function and heart function, and all cells have and need fats. Other than trans fats, which are not natural fats, your body must have the right balance of saturated fats, polyunsaturated fats and monosaturated fats along with cholesterol.

Although the polyunsaturated omega-6 fatty acids are essential for the human diet, their consumption has risen dramatically in recent years. This is related, in part, to the use of vegetable oils with high omega-6 but low omega-3 fatty acid content. Canola oil, for example, has a ratio of 66:1, and corn oil has a ratio of 12:1. This represents a major change in the American dietary pattern during the past 100 or so years. The "original" Mediterranean diet of hundreds of years ago was likely to have a ratio of about 1:1 omega-6 fatty acids and omega-3 fatty acids.

* * *

Should you lower saturated fats or total fats to reduce heart disease, and what is the evidence? Most of us were taught that we needed to eat as little fat as possible and instead eat many servings of starches such as bread, pasta, potato, and rice. Where did this advice come from?

In 1955, President Dwight Eisenhower had a heart attack. This galvanized the country because he was considered healthy, and data began to come out that heart attacks were becoming — for no apparent reason — much more common. This led to substantial anxiety. Soon fats were blamed, low fat diets were recommended, and the lost calories were replaced with multiple servings per day of carbohydrates, especially grains. The president gained weight on his low-fat diet and had six more heart attacks before he succumbed to heart disease in 1969. In retrospect, no one paid much attention to the fact that he had smoked four packs of cigarettes per day until 1949.

Actually, the critical scientific studies suggested that only saturated fats and elevated serum cholesterol are correlated with death from heart disease. None of the studies suggested that more carbohydrates were either valuable or healthy or that all fats needed to be reduced.

Nevertheless, government agencies, well-respected organizations and medical professionals began to recommend low-fat diets despite the lack of evidence that this was either appropriate or healthy. This was connected with recommendations to replace the loss in calories with carbohydrates.[32,33,34]

Now we advocate for the Mediterranean diet, which is inherently low in saturated fats and includes animal meats but in modest amounts, added sugars in negligible amounts and whole grains, not refined white flour. It emphasizes "whole foods" mostly derived from plants and mono- and polyunsaturated fats, especially olive oil and other sources of healthy fats such as fish, nuts, seeds, and avocados. The diet avoids most of today's "junk foods" (white flour, trans fats, excess omega-6 fats, salt, and sugar) as well most of the offerings at fast food restaurants.

Walter Willett, MD, a highly recognized diet expert from the Harvard School of Public Health, has described a healthy diet like this: "It's a whole package of healthy components — healthy forms of fat, whole grains compared to refined grains, a variety of fruits and vegetables, nuts, modest amounts of dairy and low amounts of red meats. Put that all together and it basically describes the Mediterranean diet."

* * *

To conclude this chapter on fats, remember that they are a fundamental and necessary part of your diet. Select healthy fats and eat them without guilt but avoid excessive saturated fats no matter the source. The long-held advice to reduce all fats and replace the lost calories with carbohydrates was in error but so, too, is the advice that saturated fats are harmless.

"Butter should not be swapped for sugar or vice versa."[35]

* * *

Consume these sources of healthy fats:

- Fin fish such as salmon, mackerel, and sardines.

- Olives and olive oil (mostly monosaturated fats).

- Coconuts and coconut oil (about 85 percent saturated fats).

- Butter — look for grass-fed organic (one-third saturated, two-thirds unsaturated).

- Nuts and seeds, especially raw.

- Avocados.

- Grass-fed meats (much more omega-3s than grain-fed but still much less than in fin fish such as salmon).

- Palm oil (50 percent saturated fat).

- Nut butters (almond, others).

- Peanut butter.

CHAPTER 16: PROTEIN

"The mind is everything. What you think you become." - Buddha

It was now nine weeks into the BOOM program. Jennifer had done well in reducing her carbohydrates, getting to the gym twice per week for the HIIT and resistance work, and walking almost every other day for about 30-40 minutes. But when her long-term boyfriend ended their relationship, she found herself needing a pastry at 9:30 in the morning, and for the first time in a long time, she went to a fast food restaurant for a cheeseburger and fries. She skipped a HIIT session. She just needed to "rebel" and escape the constraints because she was upset and rebelling, at least transiently, made her feel better and in control. But it did not last. Then she felt guilty. She was not up to the task. In her mind, she had failed.

Congratulations on coming this far, even if you are only doing one HIIT session per week and even if you are not following all of the dietary advice. Progress is about adapting, and we recognize it may take some time. Do not be discouraged if you are not able to do eight cycles of HIIT or if you have not weaned yourself off all high glycemic foods. But do not stop trying. You will get there. You will continue to increase your HIIT duration and intensity each week. Remember that finding and maintaining your healthy weight is more about your nutrition than the exercise, so put a lot of mental effort there. There will be times when you will fall off the wagon. That is okay. The next meal, the next day or whenever, just go back to eating in a low glycemic fashion with plenty of fresh, local vegetables of varying colors and textures. Include some fruits every day. Then add on the good fats like salmon, avocados, and olive oil plus the right proteins (see below). You are what you eat. Remember these two comments from Hippocrates, said more than 2,000 years ago:

"All Disease Begins in The Gut."

"If We Could Give Every Individual the Right Amount of Nourishment and Exercise – Not Too Much And Not Too Little – We Would Have Found The Safest Way To Health."

Protein

Recall that proteins are one of the three macronutrients along with carbohydrates and fats. The BOOM program encourages you to reduce your carbohydrate intake of high glycemic foods such as sugar, white flour, potatoes, and rice. Fats are fine but look to eat healthy fats. Now let us consider proteins.

Proteins are composed, in addition to carbon, hydrogen, and oxygen as in the other two macronutrients, also of nitrogen and sometimes sulfur. The proteins you eat are broken down through digestion into amino acids that can then be absorbed. The body requires amino acids to produce new proteins and replace damaged proteins. Proteins are also major components of your immune system and hormones — they are the enzymes that make all of the cellular machinery function normally. Enzymes catalyze (speed up) chemical reactions in your cells. Hormones are proteins that regulate cellular activity, including thyroid hormones or testosterone. Other proteins are used to transport various chemicals to sites in the body. Hemoglobin is a good example. It is in red blood cells and moves oxygen from the lungs to the cells in all of your organs. Proteins are the structural elements of the cells like the steel girders of a building. In short, we can say that proteins are essential for the structure,

137

regulation, and function of the human body and many different types of cells.

Once absorbed, amino acids are not stored in the body. They are either metabolized into proteins as required or excreted in the urine. Some amino acids are essential, in other words, we cannot produce them internally and we must get them from our diet. Others are "nonessential" and we can produce them from other amino acids. The term is misleading — they are all certainly critical to body function. There are twenty amino acids that can be found in the human body: nine of these are essential, seven are called "conditionally essential" because in times of stress or illness the body may not be able to make enough of them, and five are "nonessential."

Most foods contain a combination of protein, carbohydrates, and fats. Your challenge is to select foods that have a healthy combination, along the lines of what we have recommended in this book.

Many types of meat contain all of the amino acids and are called "complete" proteins. It is a common misconception that a vegetarian/vegan diet cannot provide adequate protein. Most plant-based foods (except soy and quinoa) have too little of at least one of the essential amino acids, so they are called "incomplete" proteins. But appropriate combinations of plant-based foods will be "complete." Think, for example, of rice and black beans, lintels and barley, corn and beans, pasta and peas, whole wheat bread and peanut butter, chickpeas and tahini (hummus).

Some sources of dietary protein include meat, tofu, other soy products, eggs, legumes, and dairy such as milk and cheese. We can get energy from protein because some amino acids can be converted into glucose, and as with fats, this is only done during fasting.

How much protein do you need each day? As a rule of thumb, you should consume 0.8 grams of protein per kilogram of your lean ideal body weight. Since most of us do not weigh ourselves in kilograms, just multiply your weight in pounds by 0.36. This means that if your ideal lean body weight is 160 pounds, you should consume about 58 grams of protein per day. Here is a chart of some common protein-rich foods.

Amount	Food Source	Grams of Protein
6 oz	Steak	52
3 oz	Ground beef, 90% lean/10% fat	22
4 oz	Chicken, grilled	35
6 oz	Greek yogurt, plain	18
½ cup	Cottage cheese	14
1 oz	Turkey or chicken, cooked	9
½ cup	Beans, cooked	9
1 cup	Milk	8
1 oz	Fish	7
1	Egg	6

Note that a single six-ounce steak (two decks of cards) is a full day's supply of protein. A quarter-pound hamburger provides more than one-half of the day's needs, as does a four-ounce piece of grilled chicken (about the size of the palm of your hand).

Too much protein is not healthy. Your body does not need excess, so it will either store the energy as fat, or the amino acids will be washed out in the urine. The result can be weight gain, bad breath from fermentation in the gut, constipation, diarrhea, kidney damage and other ailments. Of course, the source of the protein matters. A fatty steak from a steer finished in a stockyard eating corn and soybeans will have high concentrations of saturated fat and omega-6 fatty acids in the meat. That desired "marbling" in a prime beef roast is the fat. It makes it taste good but does not make it healthy. A steer raised entirely in the pasture on grasses has much less fat and the fats are healthier. The same can be said for sheep and chicken and for eggs from pastured hens.

Too little protein is unhealthy as well — that is the beginning of starvation. If you do not eat enough, your body will take what it needs from your muscles, which means they will lose mass and strength.

And just so you know, vegetables have some protein. Here is a chart:

Amount	Food Source	Grams of Protein
1 cup	Lima beans, cooked	12
1 cup	Soybean sprouts	9
1 cup	Green peas	7
1 cup	Spinach, kale, collards, Swiss chard, cooked	5
1 cup	Corn, cooked	5
1 cup	Asparagus, broccoli, cooked	4
1 cup	Mushrooms	4

Most fruits have some protein. For example, a cup of raspberries has 1½ grams of protein, and a cup of peaches is about the same.

Avocados are a fruit, not a vegetable, and they each have about four grams of protein.

Animal protein contains the amino acid methionine, which contains sulfur. Not all protein is metabolized and absorbed in the small intestine, and some protein reaches the large bowel where your own bacteria ferment it. This liberates hydrogen sulfide that has effects on the lining of the large bowel. It is inflammatory, mutagenic, and carcinogenic. It is what smells when you pass gas. Most gas is generated from the microbiota digestion of vegetable fiber and is carbon dioxide. Still, some is hydrogen sulfide and it smells, although this is perfectly normal and healthy if not exactly pleasant.

When you eat foods with choline (found in significant levels in red meat, egg yolks and dairy products) and L-carnitine (red meat, some energy drinks and some supplements), the microbiota digests them into trimethylamine (TMA), which is absorbed and converted in the liver to trimethylene N-oxide (TMAO). TMAO is highly inflammatory and heightens the risk for heart attacks and stroke. Does that mean you should never eat red meats? No, but as we have said repeatedly, all things in moderation. In fact, there is evidence from the Cleveland Clinic that following the Mediterranean diet helps the microbiota to not make extensive TMAO. By the way, there is a blood test for TMAO that might be worth considering. The science shows that those with the highest levels have higher rates of premature death from coronary artery disease.

The amino acid leucine, which is found in milk (human or cow), is important for the rapid growth of infants and toddlers, but we only need lots of leucine and some other amino acids at a young age when we are rapidly growing. By the way, human milk is lower in fat than cow's milk and full of maternal antibodies that provide passive immunity to the infant. Remember, no mammal except humans consume milk after weaning.

The milk industry continues to try and convince us that a large amount of milk is good for us. Our issue with milk and milk products (yogurt, ice cream, cheese, and cottage cheese) is that when consumed in daily moderate portions, they may affect the regulation of ILGF-1 (increasing cancer risk) and the mTOR aging pathway (affecting the rapidity of aging). Further, milk proteins may have immunogenic effects on the gut and, for some, galactose (one of the monosaccharides that compose lactose a disaccharide) may cause oxidative stress and contribute to fractures and a reduced lifespan.[36]

Protein is vital and essential to your diet, health, and life. The key is to select foods that have healthy proteins, eat them in moderation and do so in combination with a diet composed of a wide variety of vegetables, fruits, healthy oils, and proteins.

CHAPTER 17: INFLAMMATION – THE BASIS OF MOST CHRONIC ILLNESSES

"Let food be thy medicine and medicine be thy food." - Hippocrates

Inflammation is a normal and critical part of our body's health maintenance mechanisms. It comes to your rescue if dangerous bacteria create an infection when you get a wound or just a small cut. It protects you against cancer. Overall, it is absolutely your very good friend. Except … when it is not. Persistent inflammation, usually low grade and over time, damages various parts of your body, such as coronary blood vessels, the brain, the thyroid, joints, and the gut, and it eventually leads to disease. Typically, it's a chronic disease that cannot be cured with today's medical knowledge and will thus be with you for life.

Chronic inflammation is the basis of nearly all chronic diseases, especially the ones that cause most of the disability and death today, especially when you get older.

One hundred years ago, the most common causes of death were infectious diseases, but not today. Now it is heart disease, cancer, lung disease, stroke, and Alzheimer's disease. These are all chronic illnesses that are difficult and expensive to treat and cause substantial disability over the years. We can add obesity and diabetes mellitus to the list. Although they often do not cause death directly, they do via predisposing us to the other chronic diseases above.

The causes of chronic inflammation are legion, but a few are certainly most important. Obesity, for instance, releases chemicals into the bloodstream on a low, constant basis, and they circulate and either cause or accelerate inflammation, wherever it might be in the body. Stress does exactly the same thing. A lack of sleep follows the same pattern. Stress and sleep are generally not appreciated as major contributors to inflammation and chronic illnesses, but they truly are major contributors, and it behooves you to understand their role and work to soften their blow.

The bacteria in your gut — the microbiota — are normally your best friends and critical to good health. They can get out of kilter as a result of antibiotics and a diet that is devoid of fiber yet high in sugars and refined white flour. Now they become prime candidates to create inflammation. When unbalanced (known as dysbiosis), microbiota cause local inflammation in the intestines, create "leaky gut," and then bacteria or their byproducts, toxins in the intestines, or undigested food can enter the bloodstream where they, in turn, cause substantial inflammation.

A poor diet not only upsets the microbiota balance in your gut, it has a direct impact on inflammation as well. Our "Western diet" is typically low in vegetables and fruits with antioxidant properties and fiber, as well as healthy fats such as omega-3 fatty acids in fish or the healthy oils in avocados, nuts and seeds, and olives and olive oils. But it is high in sugars and white flour-based foods (sodas, candy, ice cream, cakes, pies, cookies, donuts, pasta, and pizza). This is just the diet that leads to inflammation. This calorie dense, nutrient lite diet means few minerals, vitamins, and other critical micronutrients.

Insulin resistance, metabolic syndrome, and diabetes (all interconnected conditions) are major accelerators of inflammation.

We have explained each of these in prior chapters, so we will not repeat here other than to remind you of their importance.

The basic message to keep in mind: You need to do whatever you can to prevent chronic inflammation from slowly but surely leading to chronic illness. A focus on a healthy diet, regular exercise, stress management, enhanced sleep, and no tobacco will be the most important steps you can take to preserve your wellness, maintain good health and avoid chronic illnesses later in life.

CHAPTER 18: SUGAR AND ARTIFICIAL SWEETENERS

"If you do what you've always done, you'll get what you always got." – Mark Twain

Jennifer never was one to put a lot of table sugar on or in her foods. But before she started the BOOM program, she did like her soda at noon, pastry during her morning coffee break (with two packets of Equal in her coffee) and a few cookies with a second soda in the later afternoon. Ice cream, though not too much, was a standard snack late in the evening. Of course, she would have some cake at a party, and she made a good apple pie with some brown sugar every now and then. Sundays were a special breakfast day, often with pancakes with real maple syrup. By keeping her food diary, she quickly realized that she actually ate a lot more sugar than she ever realized.

Sugar

Sugar plays a major role in causing obesity, metabolic syndrome, and diabetes, which in turn increases the risk of coronary artery heart disease, kidney failure, stroke, Alzheimer's disease, and other chronic illnesses. Added sugar, especially high fructose corn syrup and to a lesser degree table sugar (sucrose) and products made from refined white flour, are the major causes of metabolic syndrome and insulin resistance.

Metabolic syndrome is estimated by the CDC to affect 75 million Americans. Metabolic syndrome is defined as a person having three of the following five characteristics: high blood pressure, low HDL cholesterol (the good stuff), central obesity, elevated fasting blood sugar and high triglycerides. Metabolic syndrome is closely linked to type 2 diabetes mellitus, which along with metabolic syndrome, is a major predisposing factor to heart disease, stroke, Alzheimer's and other chronic illnesses.

We have noted previously that sugar consumption in the U.S. has increased substantially over the years and is now 50 percent higher than in the 1920s. Although the American Heart Association recommends men should limit their added sugar to 36 grams per day (or less than nine teaspoons per day), most men consume far more than these recommendations. Sugar has four calories per gram, so 36 grams means 144 calories — more sugar means more calories. The number for women is 25 grams per day (or six teaspoons), which equates to 100 calories per day. Women also consume far more than the recommendation.

A can of soda has 39 grams or 156 calories, a Cinnabon has 14 teaspoons of sugar (or 55 grams or 220 calories), a small Snickers bar has 30 grams (or five teaspoons) and a cookie, depending on size, has about 18 grams or five teaspoons of sugar.

Artificial Sweeteners

Artificial sweeteners include NutraSweet or Equal, which have the chemical name aspartame; Splenda, also known as sucralose; Sweet'N Low, also known as saccharin; and Sweet-1 or acesulfame-k. Sugar Twin, or cyclamate, was banned in the United States years ago, but it is still available in Canada.

There are some other sweeteners, especially in gum, such as Z-sweet, which is known as erythritol. This is naturally found in pears, melons, and grapes and recently has been found to have some antioxidant activity. It is absorbed in the intestine and does not have any laxative effect like its sister compounds — xylitol and sorbitol. Truvia, or stevia, comes from the stevia plant and is thought to be a natural compound.

The latter two are probably harmless, at least according to current information. We will focus on the first group because these are among the most-used food additives.

One might think that, when trying to attain a healthy weight, it would be beneficial to use these noncaloric sweeteners. Unfortunately, this is far from the truth. Artificial sweeteners have no nutritional value. The "good" of them is that they contain no calories, so as a substitute for sugar, they could be beneficial. But the most important "bad" is that substituting a sweet taste for actual sugar only continues the addiction to sweetness. You need to train your brain's pleasure center to no longer demand sweet. That is one of the most important concepts in the BOOM program.

Another negative of artificial sweeteners is thinking, "Well, I drank a diet soda, so now it must be okay to have that piece of cake." Not so — the cake includes sugar and the flour digests into sugar. And another negative is that these sweeteners may limit your tolerance for more complex flavors, causing you to shun healthy foods.

Of increasing concern is that they have an adverse impact on the microbiome. The common artificial sweeteners are related to the onset of insulin resistance, glucose intolerance and ultimately metabolic syndrome and diabetes, probably in part by causing changes in the colonic microbiota. Animal experiments show that the negative impact can be transferred to germ-free mice by fecal transplants from the affected mice. In short, artificial sweeteners lead to a dysbiosis (or an abnormal, deleterious change) of the intestinal microbiota.[37]

A large "multiethnic study of atherosclerosis" found that daily diet drinks, when compared to none, were correlated with a 36 percent increased relative risk of metabolic syndrome (for 478 people among 2,288 or 21 percent versus 129 people among 501 or 26 percent). Diet drinks were correlated with a 67 percent increased relative risk of type 2 diabetes mellitus (for 221 people among 2,961 or 7 percent compared to 75 people among 681 or 11 percent).[38]

This is also a good time to indicate that "relative risk" is not the same as absolute risk, which is why we entered all the numbers. Yes, diet drinks were associated with a 36 percent increased relative risk, but that is based on the absolute risks of 21 percent versus 26 percent. You have to decide if that is a difference worth your concern. We would say "yes" because it is one more indication that artificial sweeteners have much more of an adverse impact on health than ever previously considered.

The neurobiology of artificial sweeteners in the brain is also fascinating. Upon placing artificially sweetened beverages or food in your mouth, this sweet flavor is detected instantaneously by the taste buds on the tongue. The tongue receptors send messages to the brain immediately. The brain then believes there is incoming sugar, and a cascade of events happen that increase neurotransmitters in your brain and make you hungry. In addition, the brain signals the digestive system to get ready for incoming calories. However, there are no calories coming, so your hunger persists. The hunger could be satiated if you started to absorb calories, but there are none. The calories would increase your basal insulin levels and your leptin levels, which would then quell your hunger — that is if you are not leptin resistant from being overweight or obese.

Our recommendation is to use real sugar in moderation, if at all, rather than use artificial sweeteners. They may have some value in reducing calories, but they are certainly not a panacea and their negative health impacts are real.

Think of it like this:

- Trying to lose/maintain weight? Eat less sugar!
- Trying to avoid diabetes and coronary artery disease? Eat less sugar!
- Artificial sweeteners are a poor crutch!

Yes, sugar is killing us, but artificial sweeteners are not the way to save your life.

CHAPTER 19: SUPPLEMENTS

"You cannot expect to hit the jackpot if you don't put a few nickels in the machines." - Flip Wilson

The vitamin supplement business is a multi-billion-dollar enterprise. If you are going to take vitamins and supplements, it is important that you are knowledgeable about the risks, benefits, indications, and possible side effects of these over-the-counter drugs. It is crucial that you use a quality product that will not interact with an existing condition or prescription medication.

Here are some of our recommendations. Keep in mind that recommendations are based on the best information at hand and are subject to change. We have made every effort to base these recommendations on the latest published, peer-reviewed scientific information. Vitamins and supplements should be respected and taken for a specific purpose, not because crazy cousin Eddie says it helps. And very importantly, they are *supplements*, which are to be adjuncts to your lifestyle efforts to eat a well-rounded nourishing diet on an everyday basis. No pill can replace a sensible well-rounded diet, nor can they balance a lack of exercise, excess chronic stress, or inadequate sleep.

Multivitamins

Yes, for just about everyone. Many people take a multivitamin each day, but until recently, there was no convincing evidence that this was necessary provided you were eating a quality diet. Newer data, however, suggests that a multivitamin from a quality manufacturer is of real value.[39]

Vitamin D

Yes, for just about everybody. Try to get 2,000 units of vitamin D-3 per day. Vitamin D is not just important for your bones; it helps strengthen your immune system and has a multitude of activities in many organs and systems.

We think getting direct sunlight is important as well. About twenty minutes a day increases the conversion of inactive vitamin D-2 to active vitamin D-3 and the production of nitric oxide, a powerful vasodilator. A worthwhile read is this controversial article which may be heralding a new view about the value of direct sun exposure: "Is sunscreen the new margarine?"[40]

You probably think of vitamin D as the vitamin needed to prevent rickets and that just a small amount is necessary, but vitamin D in larger amounts is necessary for nearly every tissue in your body. It is the normal product of sun exposure to your uncovered skin. Vitamin D depletion or deficiency can increase when sunlight is diminished, such as in late fall and winter. Actually, most people living in temperate climates get too little sunlight-activated vitamin D. The combination of clouds, rain, shorter days, and clothes that cover most of the body all impact sunlight exposure. Moreover, today we use sunscreens to protect us from skin cancer, so even exposed skin cannot convert vitamin D. Typically, older Americans get less sunlight. Additionally, if you are overweight or darker, your risk for vitamin D deficiency is significant.

Low levels of vitamin D can contribute to osteoporosis. Epidemiologic studies suggest higher rates of colon, breast and prostate cancer may be related to low vitamin D levels. There is also a higher rate of autoimmune diseases such as multiple sclerosis, rheumatoid arthritis, and type 1 diabetes in patients with low vitamin D levels. Profound reductions in vitamin D can cause muscle weakness, fatigue, and aching, which can be misdiagnosed as fibromyalgia. Decreased cardiac function and increased blood pressure have also been associated with low vitamin D levels. Vitamin D may even keep you from getting influenza (flu).[41] The accepted recommended blood level has risen in recent years, as new data emerged on the importance of vitamin D in these many metabolic functions. In short, everyone needs to be sure they have adequate circulating vitamin D levels. There is a simple blood test available.

But, as in much of medicine, there is some controversy about the acceptable lower level of vitamin D. Some feel 12.5, others 20, still others (all highly reputable) suggest 30-60 ng/ml of blood serum. Your doctor may be as confused as everyone else. The good news is there is general agreement that the higher levels are certainly not deleterious. So, get the blood test and talk it over with your provider. Here are interesting articles in the *New England Journal of Medicine*.[42,43] We believe 40 or greater is a good goal.

There are numerous vitamin D supplements. If you start a vitamin D supplement, be sure that it is vitamin D-3, also known as cholecalciferol. Multivitamins generally do not have an adequate amount of vitamin D, and you will probably be told to take 2,000-5,000 units per day.

Curcumin

Maybe, it depends on your situation. The polyphenol curcumin is one of the ingredients in the spice turmeric, which gives curry its yellow color. It has powerful anti-inflammatory effects. It is consumed heavily in India where, incidentally, they have one of the lowest rates of Alzheimer's in the world. According to a recent review, curcumin is useful to aid oxidation and inflammation, metabolic syndrome, arthritis, anxiety, and elevated lipids. They indicate that a low dose may be of general health benefit to apparently healthy individuals to help maintain wellness.[44] A daily dose would be 500 mg to 1,000 mg per day. Be certain that any product you purchase has black pepper in the formulation. Curcumin is poorly absorbed from the gut into the bloodstream, and black pepper contains piperine, a natural substance that inhibits the breakdown of curcumin, which enhances curcumin in the blood by 2,000 percent.[45]

Omega-3 Fatty Acids

Maybe. Omega-3 fatty acids (O3FAs) are known as essential fatty acids because your cells need them but cannot make them from the nutrients you eat, so you must consume them directly. They are among the polyunsaturated fatty acids and are created by certain plants, especially algae, which in turn are eaten by fish and then eaten by you. Some plants such as flax have a modest amount of omega-3s, especially ALA, but your cellular machinery does not convert it quickly to other important fatty acids, so flax meal alone is not sufficient for your needs. Interestingly, if you look at the rate of sudden death in the United States versus Japan, it is strikingly different: sudden death rates in Japan are one-fifth compared to the U.S. Could it be because the Japanese have high O3FA blood levels? The answer appears to be "yes," at least in part. The best source of O3FA is wild caught salmon, but most any cold-water fin fish has a good amount. Try for two to three servings per week. Unfortunately, that is well above what most Americans consume today. Indeed, the American diet is generally deficient in O3FAs.

Two supplement options exist — fish oil capsules and capsules of DHA/EPA derived from algae. The value of supplements of O3FAs is controversial. Reports at the American Heart Association meeting in November 2018 and concurrently published in the *New England*

Journal of Medicine gave conflicting results. One trial showed that marine-based capsules (1 gram per day) in healthy individuals had no effect in lowering later heart disease.[46] Another study of only individuals with high triglycerides but statin-controlled LDL indicated that a high dose (4 grams of purified EPA) did decrease heart disease deaths.[47]

What to make of this? First, remember that no supplement can top a good diet. But perhaps there is utility in taking a dose of about 1 gram (1,000 mg) per day of either formulation as there is no apparent recognized adverse effects.

Probiotics and Prebiotics

Probably not and maybe. Remember from Chapter 13, prebiotics are the food sources that the healthy bacteria in your colon love and indeed need to survive and thrive – and then aid your health. Prebiotic foods are largely those with high levels of fiber content such as many vegetables and fruits. It is the fiber that the bacteria utilize as energy sources. Probiotics are living microorganisms found in fermented foods like sauerkraut and yogurt.

You are what you eat! If you take in adequate prebiotics (over 30 grams fiber per day) in your foods and a few servings per week of probiotic foods, there may be little or no need to take supplements.

Vitamin K-2

Maybe. Vitamin K is a group of related compounds, including K1 and K2. The former is found in dark greens especially. The latter is in meats, cheeses and eggs and the Japanese soy-based fermented product called natto and is synthesized by your intestinal bacteria. K-2 is an important fat-soluble vitamin that protects your heart and brain and moves calcium out of the blood into the bone.[48] Vitamin K-2 may be worthwhile to take for better bones, and some studies suggest it is valuable for decreasing cardiovascular disease risk. The usual dose assumed appropriate for adults is 90-120 micrograms per day, and supplements are available in 100 mcg formulations.

Calcium

No, for most people. For many years, the conventional advice from physicians was to take calcium tablets to prevent osteoporosis and cardiac events since supplemental calcium was found to bring down blood pressure by a few points, though that effect seems to wear off after a couple of months of daily use.

Unfortunately, the logic did not prove correct. As it turns out, from large-scale studies, including the Woman's Health Care Initiative, women who took calcium supplements had more cardiac events than those who did not. Daily supplemental calcium seems to spike calcium levels in the blood, increasing the risk of blood clotting, as well as lead to calcification and plaque thickness in the coronary arteries. So, the current recommendation is to get your calcium from the food you eat. What an outstanding idea! For an interesting video on this topic, see this endnote.[49]

Baby Aspirin and Full-Strength Aspirin

Yes, for some people, no, for some, and maybe, for others. Patients with existing cardiovascular disease may be good candidates to take daily aspirin, often 81 mg or "baby aspirin." This is called "secondary prevention" since it is aimed at protecting from a second occurrence. The recommendation is based on the Second International Study of Infarct Survival (ISIS-2), which found that giving aspirin to patients with myocardial infarction within 24 hours of presentation led to a significant reduction in later cardiovascular deaths. What about taking aspirin if you are healthy for primary prevention, especially if you have risk factors for heart disease such as diabetes, hypertension, hyperlipidemia, and/or a family history of premature heart disease? This has been a somewhat controversial but commonly followed recommendation. There was a recent meta-analysis in the *Journal of the American Medical Association*.[50] Among 164,225 individuals who did not have heart disease, aspirin use led to a lower risk of cardiac events and deaths but an increased risk of bleeding. The accompanying editorial suggested that aspirin could be valuable but that a program of comprehensive risk factor reduction, including lifestyle modifications to actually reduce the risk of disease, was preferential.[51] We recommend a thoughtful discussion with your physician before taking aspirin daily.

As for cancer, in one study, aspirin users had a 48 percent reduction in the odds of developing pancreatic cancer compared with non-users. The benefits existed for the use of low and regular strength aspirin, and the risk of pancreatic cancer decreased as the number of years of aspirin use increased. The Harvard Women's Study also demonstrated a 20 percent reduction in risk of colon cancer for women but no difference in polyp formation after taking daily aspirin for many years.

Aspirin is not without its drawbacks, including gastrointestinal bleeding and ulcer formation. Both occurred slightly more often among women in the study taking aspirin. Gastrointestinal bleeding was 8.3 percent in the aspirin group and 7.3 percent in the placebo group, and ulcer formation was 7.3 percent in the aspirin group, 6.2 percent in the placebo group.

For many adults, the benefits of taking a single dose of baby aspirin on a daily basis outweigh the risks. But a recent study called Aspree questioned if this advice was also appropriate for older individuals. The study asked if the potential benefits of low-dose aspirin to reduce heart disease, stroke, some cancers, and dementia outweigh the risks, especially bleeding, in healthy people over age 70. The answer was there were no advantages but some disadvantages with bleeding.[52]

Francis Collins, MD, the director of the National Institutes of Health, recently wrote this after the conclusion of the Aspree study: "For older people now taking aspirin, ... consult with your doctor ... it appears that if you're a healthy older person with no history of cardiovascular disease, an aspirin a day may not have the potential we once thought to keep the doctor away."[53]

But another study published around the same time looked at whether the 81 mg dose of aspirin was suitable for everyone. They found that low-dose aspirin was only effective in older patients who weighed less than about 150 pounds. That excluded a very large number of potential beneficiaries. So, they concluded, a "one-dose-fits-all" approach to aspirin is unlikely to be optimal, at least for older individuals.[54]

There seem to be no clear-cut answers, so if your doctor or nurse practitioner is confused, so is everyone else. Aspirin is indicated for most people who have had a heart attack or other clear evidence of coronary artery disease. The risk of bleeding is low, but the real benefit of aspirin in low doses as primary prevention is questionable, especially for individuals who are heavier.

Antioxidants

Maybe but probably not. Vitamins A, C, E, Coenzyme Q plus selenium, copper and zinc all are either direct antioxidants or assist antioxidant enzymes function. Yes, antioxidant supplements are readily available, but first consider that nutrient-dense foods are heavy with naturally containing antioxidants. These allow the body to naturally combat oxidation and the production of free radicals.

Oxidation is a normal process in your cells, and part of that natural process is to quell excess oxidation so it cannot cause cellular harm. But there are many things you can do to accentuate oxidation, such as smoking, sitting, not sleeping, eating the wrong foods, and experiencing out-of-control stress. We recommend that you aggressively work on lifestyle modifications rather than rely on a pill as a crutch. Instead, eat nutrient-dense, calorie lite foods with abandon, get your stress under control, get a good night's sleep, and get regular exercise. You will feel better and you will save some money.

In regard to Coenzyme Q 10, we do believe if you are taking a statin drug it is worth it to also take this antioxidant, as it is well accepted that statins deplete your Coenzyme Q 10 reserve, which may contribute to muscle aches that are a frequent complaint of those taking a statin. The best preparation to use is the active reduced form of Coenzyme Q 10, or ubiquinol 100 mg per day.

Dark Chocolate

Yes. Dark chocolate is also a good source of antioxidants and has a number of healthy properties, such as improving blood flow, lowering blood pressure, reducing heart disease risks, lowering bad LDL, increasing good HDL, helping brain function and creating a sense of happiness just to have a taste! So, if you are finishing up your day and have a craving, have a small serving of dark chocolate — preferably 85 percent cocoa. It was found that dark chocolate has antidepressant effects, and a small amount may decrease the likelihood of depression.[55] Milk chocolate should be avoided for two reasons: the sugar content is something you do not need, and the dairy products in milk chocolate negate the positive effects of dark chocolate. For migraine sufferers, dark chocolate contains vasoactive ingredients, and too much can, in susceptible people, stimulate a migraine, so be careful.

* * *

By way of background, beginning in the mid-1990s, Dr. Oken became involved in omega-3 fatty acid clinical research. Later, he became a part-time consultant for a nutritional company. In the process, he met Dr. Julian Bailes. At the time, Dr. Bailes was chairman of the Department of Neurosurgery at the West Virginia University School of Medicine and was studying the effect of omega-3 fatty acids as a remedy for brain trauma. Dr. Bailes gained national attention when he treated Randy McCloy, the lone survivor of the Sago Mine accident. Part of his treatment was high-dose omega-3 fatty acids. McCloy made an astonishing near-miraculous recovery that made headline news. Dr. Bailes' work on repetitive head trauma led to him playing a central role in approaching the National Football League about the dangers of head trauma. (Alec Baldwin plays him in the movie *Concussion*.)

Dr. Oken is also on the scientific advisory board of Persona Nutrition. The board advises the company based on the most recent evidence-based science. The company has a computer-driven algorithm that allows the user to get advice about the best supplements to use based on current medications, medical history, and current medical issues. Supplements should be carefully used and periodically reassessed for need. Those with an excellent diet likely do not need supplements, according to our colleague Dr. Michael Roizen, the inventor of RealAge and head of wellness at Cleveland Clinic. He comments, "Since more than 90 percent of those taking the nutrition test at RealAge.com [it is free] do not get recommended amounts of one or another vitamin or mineral in their diet, we think half a multi twice a day is a great inexpensive insurance policy against an imperfect diet."

CHAPTER 20: WATER AND ALCOHOL AND FOOD SHOPPING

"Don't find fault with a remedy." - Henry Ford

Jennifer had always followed the rule of drinking a fair amount of water before exercising and sometimes kept a bottle of water with her to sip on as she exercised, whether or not she felt thirsty.

Water, Water Everywhere.

Let us go over some important and rather surprising information about water.

First, water is your preferred beverage. Do not drink extra calories with your meals. Water is the #1 nutrient for your body. If you are dehydrated, it can definitely affect how you feel — sleepy, sluggish, foggy, slow, even confused. Your brain rapidly reacts to this since it is 75 percent water. The remedy, of course, is rehydration, and it starts within five minutes and peaks at twenty minutes after drinking the water you need. Cool water is absorbed about 20 percent faster than body temperature water.[56]

Chronically dehydrated people are at higher risk for kidney stones, bladder cancer, and heart disease, to name but a few. How much water do you need? Studies suggest women need four to seven cups of water and men need six to eleven cups per day.

Does tea count or is it dehydrating due to the perceived diuretic effect? The great thing about tea is that it is full of antioxidants, especially green tea and black tea, but if it causes dehydration, that is not good. Despite various commentaries to the contrary, there is no evidence that tea has a significant diuretic effect, so there is no concern that it will dehydrate you.

One of the greatest medical remedies ever discovered was that water and salt and sugar in the right ratio could save the lives of children with cholera and other diarrheal illness in developing countries. This has saved hundreds of millions of lives. This led to the notion that oral rehydration with sports drinks and or coconut water is superior to plain old water. Not so — there is no evidence that these are superior to good old water. Sports drinks are loaded with sugar, and it is like drinking a soda. However, potassium replacement can be helpful if you are dehydrated from excessive sweating. Consider coconut water with a significant concentration of potassium but beware if you have kidney disease as the potassium levels can rise to dangerous heights.

When you exercise, should you water load? No! There is no scientific basis behind the saying of "Don't wait until you feel thirsty to drink." Drinking too much before or during exercise can lead to low sodium levels in your bloodstream, called hyponatremia. For those involved in strenuous exercise such as marathon running, this can lead to illness and even death.

Your body is smart, and it tells you when to drink, so drink when you are thirsty. Let thirst be your guide!

* * *

Alcohol – Enjoyable in limited quantities.

There are many social occasions when people come together to enjoy wine, beer, and cocktails. The notion that a glass of red wine per day is healthy from a medicinal standpoint is controversial. We do know that the polyphenols in red wine have antioxidant value. Resveratrol (an antioxidant in red grapes) increases the lifespan in mice, but the equivalent amount that would presumably be needed in humans far exceeds the amount in one glass of red wine (2 mg). There is presently no clear scientific evidence that large doses of resveratrol (500 to 1,000 mg) is beneficial.

There are lots of reasons to limit alcohol, especially while working toward a leaner weight. Alcohol is an empty calorie, and there is little if any nutritional value. Consumption may affect your sleep by causing drowsiness as well as frequent night awakenings, ultimately having a negative effect on your sleep cycle. There is some debate as to whether it affects fat burning, and at seven calories per gram, it may be burned for energy first, thus inhibiting the body's ability to access fat stores. Excessive intake can contribute to fatty accumulation in your liver (alcoholic fatty liver disease). Also, remember that obesity causes fatty liver as well (nonalcoholic fatty liver disease, or NAFLD). NAFLD has surpassed alcoholic liver disease and hepatitis C as the top cause of cirrhosis (scarring and contraction of the liver) in the United States.

Drinking alcohol during a meal can affect digestion and lead to poorer nutrient absorption, diarrhea and exacerbated irritable bowel syndrome. Daily moderate consumption does increase the risk for all cancers, especially GI cancers. Even a small amount of daily drinking in women is associated with a small yet significant increase in the risk for breast cancer. The possibility that light daily drinking may decrease cardiovascular disease is supported by published studies[57], but if you are trying to get healthy, you are better off minimizing consumption.

Bottom line, enjoy but minimize.

* * *

Shopping for food should be fun, but it can also be expensive. Let us pull together the recommendations scattered throughout this book.

Vegetables and fruits are best if they are locally grown, naturally ripe and organic, not subjected to pesticides or herbicides. But realistically, today many products are grown thousands of miles away and shipped by truck. This means that they are picked many days before they are ripe so they will remain firm and not bruised over the period of shipping. Organic products are usually more expensive than conventional, and other than for residual pesticides and herbicides, are probably not any healthier. Fortunately, many organic items are only marginally more expensive today as more farmers convert to organic production. Here, then, are a few suggestions.

Try to avoid the "dirty dozen" grown conventionally. According to the Environmental Working Group, which uses data from the Department of Agriculture, these are the twelve most frequently found to have residual pesticides in 2018.[58] Of course, whether organic or not, you should always wash before preparing for meals.

Dirty Dozen Foods
Frequently found to have
residual Pesticides

1. Strawberries
2. Spinach
3. Nectarines
4. Apples
5. Grapes
6. Peaches
7. Cherries
8. Pears
9. Tomatoes
10. Celery
11. Potatoes
12. Sweet Bell Peppers

164

These the Clean Fifteen for 2018, which are produce items that tended to have the least pesticide residues:

Clean Fifteen Foods
Infrequently found to have residual Pesticides

1. Avocados
2. Sweet Corn
3. Pineapples
4. Cabbage
5. Onions
6. Sweet Frozen Peas
7. Papayas
8. Asparagus
9. Mangos
10. Eggplant
11. Honeydew Melon
12. Kiwi
13. Cantaloupe
14. Cauliflower
15. Broccoli

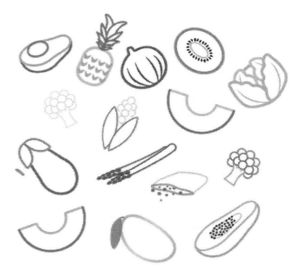

If you want to buy items that ripened on the tree or the vine, consider your local farmer's market, at least during the growing season in your area. It is interesting that products destined for freezing are harvested at the time of peak ripeness and flash frozen, so often a frozen product will be tastier than fresh from the grocery. The same cannot be said for canned foods since they often have high levels of added salt.

Most fish in the market today are farm raised. As a general rule, farm raised fish are less expensive than their wild caught brethren. In that regard, farm raised has been a boon for shoppers' wallets. Let us use salmon as an example since salmon is such a standard because of its high levels of omega-3 fatty acids. In nature, the salmon swims out to sea, eats algae loaded with omega-3s, and after a few years, swims back to its birthplace upriver. During the migration upriver, the fish are caught with their highest concentration of healthy fats and large, strong muscles. Farm raised are kept in a restricted area and fed foods, usually other fish byproducts that include omega-3 fatty acids, resulting in fish that also have a high concentration of these fats. Which is healthier? It is controversial. We prefer wild caught. But if you are going to buy farm raised (of any type of fish), be sure you buy from a reputable fishmonger who can tell you exactly where that fish was raised and how it was raised. Frankly, many types of fish from farms in developing countries are questionable.

Most beef in the store comes from steers that were raised on the range initially and then sent to feeding pens near the slaughterhouse. There they remain in cramped conditions for a few months, eating corn and soybeans all day, rapidly adding fat to their muscle. In contrast, cattle that graze on local grasses not only have less fat but also healthier fat with more omega-3s and less omega-6s. After grain feeding, the ratio switches to almost all omega-6s and very little omega-3s plus saturated fats. We recommend beef (and lamb) that is grass-fed throughout life. It is much healthier but certainly more expensive and harder to find. You, of course, could argue that since our recommendation is also to eat a card deck-size portion of red meat only once a week or so, that maybe the fat content of the meat is less relevant than if you were consuming many beef or lamb meals per week.

Poultry has the same issue. Most chickens are raised in cramped conditions indoors until slaughter. Even organic chickens are usually raised in the same quarters. Chicken is much tastier if the birds are able to go outside and peck in the ground. Laying hens usually live full-time in small cages, never seeing the light of day or getting a chance to exercise. Look for free-range chicken and eggs, preferably raised organically.

A good general rule: Avoid the middle aisles of the grocery store since they are loaded with processed foods. If you must purchase there, read the labels carefully. We like Michael Pollen's admonition:

If it has more than five ingredients or has ingredients whose names you have never heard of or cannot pronounce, move on. Be aware that the meat and produce sections increasingly have processed food mixed in with the "plain" meat or produce.

In the dairy aisle, look for yogurt that has "live active cultures." As a general rule, those with added flavors or fruits also have added sugars and do not have live cultures. Milk and milk products from organically fed cows are becoming more prevalent, but being organic does not necessarily mean that the cows were grass range-fed. They could be held in large barns and fed with organic materials but rarely see the light of day.

Yes, organic vegetables and fruits are more expensive. Grass-fed meats and wild caught fish are more expensive. And so, too, are organic dairy products. On the other hand, you will be saving by not buying sodas, ice cream, cakes, cookies, and other junk foods. Consider all the options and then do what makes the most sense for you and your wallet.

It was time for Jennifer to go back to see her primary care physician. She told him about keeping the food diary, reducing her carbs, avoiding sweets and artificial sweeteners, increasing her vegetables, including lots of dark leafy greens and other veggies of many colors, along with healthy fats, especially fish and olive oil. She described the HIIT exercises and how she ate nothing after supper and not again until about two hours after finishing the morning HIIT exercise. She told him that she took daily 30-minute walks and twice a week did resistance exercises at the gym after finishing HIIT. She was sleeping better now that she turned off her cell phone early, kept the room quiet and dark and went to bed earlier than before. Now she was getting about 7 ½ hours of sleep. She had started a yoga class at the gym and was doing some meditation most days at home. She also told him about what happened with her boyfriend and described her interaction with her boss and how work was much less stressful.

She got good news from her doctor. Her weight was down (she knew that, of course), as was her belly circumference. But in addition, her blood pressure was now normal, her cholesterol levels were fine, and there was no evidence of insulin resistance. Her physician was proud of her and said so. He said she was his poster child for what attention to lifestyle could mean. She had done what was needed — of course, she would have to stick with it — and proved that the combination of diet, exercise, stress management, and enhanced sleep would alleviate many of the conditions that lead to inflammation and ultimately chronic illnesses.

CHAPTER 21: EXERCISE AND YOUR BRAIN

"We don't stop playing because we grow old. We grow old because we stop playing." - George Bernard Shaw

You have undoubtedly felt a pickup in energy and mood after exercise. It feels good and actually helps to create a desire to repeat your workout next time. It does not need to be a BOOM-type workout. Even a pleasant walk for a half-hour or so will give you that mental boost.

What is happening? A lot. That sense of increased energy, mood and attention is very real. It relates to the immediate release of neuroactive chemicals, including serotonin, dopamine, and norepinephrine. These circulate to brain cells but also to the rest of your body. The effects last for a few hours. You will also notice an increased ability to focus your attention, and your reaction time — how quickly you hit the brakes — goes up as well. These will last but a few hours, but it is striking that just a simple walk, preferably a walk that raises your heart rate, will have such a profound impact on your mental capacities.

Regular exercise has even more profound effects on your brain and these changes are long term. Two critical areas of the brain are the prefrontal cortex, where your "executive functions" lie, and the hippocampus, which is critical for memory function. Regular exercise leads to the development of new brain neurons and concurrently new pathways among the brain circuits. Repetitive exercise allows the prefrontal cortex to increase its attentive function. The hippocampus and the prefrontal cortex both actually enlarge, as can be measured with something called volumetric MRI scans. These new neurons in the hippocampus and cortex impact the ability to increase long-term memory. Remember from the earlier chapter about sleep how the hippocampus chooses items to be placed in long-term memory in the cortex. This is a critical function and depends on adequate neuronal capacity in both areas.

Although just that 30-minute walk will have a positive impact on hippocampus enlargement (along with being a pleasant time to "clear" your brain with the sounds and the smell of the air), doing the HIIT exercise will dramatically speed the process. Do both over the course of the week!

By exercising, you create a protective effect for your brain. These two critical areas are the first to be damaged by age and by neurodegenerative diseases such as Alzheimer's. An enlarged hippocampus and an enlarged prefrontal cortex mean that there is more reserve, and some damage will not have as dramatic an impact on cognitive function. You could think of exercise as storing away a brain reserve for your elder years, just as an IRA does with money. Start early in adulthood and the impact builds up over the years and, just like that IRA, the investment compounds. Remember, exercise is free — there is no charge for this prescription.

Jennifer had her ups and downs, but she stuck with the BOOM program, and at the end of twelve weeks, she could easily do the eight cycles of HIIT, no longer had a strong craving for sweets, was sleeping better and was less stressed. Her daily diet included lots of simply prepared vegetables plus various healthy fats, including fish twice per week, avocados, olive oil on her salads, olives and some nuts or seeds most days. She had beef or chicken occasionally, about the size of a deck of cards. She still kept to a low carbohydrate diet but not limited to 50 grams per day. She even rejoined her pizza crowd on Friday night. Over the twelve weeks, she had lost fifteen pounds.

And one year later, Jennifer maintained the Mediterranean diet with limited carbs, still did the HIIT exercise twice weekly along with resistance exercises, walked daily, was sleeping well for about 7 ½ hours per night and felt generally energetic and content. She found that keeping to the time-restricted eating of nothing after supper and, on HIIT days, nothing until about two hours after exercise, was not difficult, uncomfortable nor stressful. Her weight was now down by a total of forty pounds since she had begun. She felt good, and looking in the mirror, she felt proud of herself. She also had a new boyfriend. Life was good.

She invited Ellen to join her for lunch at the sushi restaurant by the waterfront. This had become a favorite. This was a special lunch. It was a "Thank You" to Ellen for being so direct, honest, and yet helpful the year before. It had made a huge difference in her life.

CHAPTER 22: SOME THOUGHTS FOR SENIORS

"Some guy said to me: Don't you think you're too old to sing rock 'n' roll? I said: You'd better check with Mick Jagger." - Cher

Jennifer is 45, about the average age of those who enter the BOOM program with Dr. Oken. Some are younger and some are older, but what about those who are decidedly seniors, probably retired, a bit or more overweight, now noticing that they are indeed older with some diminishment of vision, hearing, mobility or even cognition? Does BOOM have a place in their lives? The answer is a resounding "yes." It is never too late to begin. Here is another composite person, one that Dr. Schimpff often encounters at the retirement community where he and his wife have lived for the past four years:

Dave is 75 and feels that he is in generally good health but can clearly see the impact of his years. He is gray now, has wrinkles in his skin, has cataracts, and finds conversation in a crowded restaurant difficult. He is particularly discouraged that when he looks in the mirror, he sees a real diminishment of muscle mass, and he knows that his strength is lower. His balance is okay, but he notices that he has to "catch" himself more frequently now. And, truth be told, his memory is not what it was. He and his wife have lived in the retirement community of 2,000 with its six restaurants, huge pool, fitness center, all sorts of opportunities for social interaction and continued lifelong learning for about two years. Over that time, he has gained about eight pounds or so, and he can see it in his belly. It seems there is a saying among residents that everyone gains weight after moving in. Dave is concerned that he will continue to "lose ground" in the coming years with more muscle loss, more balance problems, less energy, and less stamina. He wonders if there is anything he can do to slow or even reverse the process. And he is especially concerned that he might develop dementia — he sees many residents in the early stages and knows that when it progresses, they will lose their independence and move to another building for care.

Dave is a prime candidate for BOOM. He can eat healthy meals in his retirement community. He can use the fitness center and the pool. He can take walks outside or, in inclement weather, can walk for more than a mile through the main corridors. There is on-site yoga, Tai Chi and massage to help with stress. He will need to consider meditation and adjusting his habits around bedtime. He and his wife can do the BOOM program together, which will give them the added boost of positive reinforcement. Of course, he absolutely needs to check with his primary care physician to be sure there is nothing in the BOOM program that would be deleterious to his health. With personal trainers in the fitness center, he can get help starting HIIT.

As part of the community concept, everyone receives a meal per day in one of the restaurants. The daily meal allows one to choose a soup, a salad, an entrée, two sides, a dessert, and a beverage. The menus are extensive, they change seasonally, and there are always three specials each week. There are healthy choices but plenty of opportunities for the less healthy. Seniors need fewer calories than when they were younger, and their gut absorbs fewer nutrients than before. They need a diet heavy with nutrients in order to get enough but lite in calories. That concept is not well understood by most, so they continue to eat as always and wonder why they gain weight. Given an extensive menu, it takes some willpower but also some understanding to choose wisely.

Our suggestion to Dave would be for he and his wife to take that meal at midday rather than the evening. Invite friends to join in a few days each week to ensure social engagement. Choose a healthy salad, one with dark leafy greens and some chopped veggies on top with olive oil and vinegar for a dressing. Select the fish entrée, either grilled or poached and without sauces. Do not order the chicken breaded and fried. Select two vegetables steamed or sautéed and avoid the potatoes au gratin, the creamed spinach and certainly the macaroni and cheese. Decline the rolls and butter. Skip the dessert, even the ones made with artificial sweeteners. A fresh fruit plate would be fine. Have water with lemon, an unsweetened iced tea or black coffee but not a diet soda. Dave will leave the table comfortably full and have had an opportunity to interact with others. For supper in their apartment, they can consider a few veggies of different types and colors each cooked simply and differently — steamed, baked, stir-fried. And do not forget, nothing after supper until breakfast the next day.

Dave will need to include a thirty-minute walk every day. He should avoid prolonged sitting and move around. He should follow a good diet according to the concepts presented previously, such as eating his major meal by early afternoon, with nothing after supper and continuing to mid-morning, to allow the body to work its overnight magic of rest and restoration. HIIT twice weekly in the morning will help increase growth hormone levels, and by not eating before or for a few hours after, the GH levels can stay up and maintain and build muscle mass. Resistance exercises twice weekly will likewise help to preserve muscle mass and strength. Adding in some balance exercises would be an additional benefit. Dealing with the stresses of life is critical, as is a good night's sleep. And although not mentioned as part of the BOOM program, continued intellectual challenges in the senior years and social engagement are important for maintaining brain health, as are diet, exercise, stress reduction, and sleep. Here is an added bonus from the HIIT approach: If Dave was to get an MRI of his brain with a measurement of the volume of his hippocampus, he might be pleasantly surprised six months later to learn it had substantially enlarged while following the BOOM program.

The advantages of the BOOM program make sense for just about everyone. Of course, most seniors do not live in a retirement community with all of the options available. For those living at home, you can just follow the BOOM program as outlined in the previous chapters using a gym for your HIIT and resistance weight training. Remember, it is never too late to get started, and you will be glad you did.

BOOM! Recap:

- Log your food since you eat more than you think.

- Try to keep your net carbohydrate count less than 50 grams per day. Net carbs = Total carbs - fiber grams, but if you are trying to reset your pleasure center, keep total carbs less than 50 grams per day for a week.

- Do your HIIT fasting, except for coffee, water, or tea.

- Try not to eat for at least two hours after exercise.

- Do not just think it, say it out loud: "I am not going to eat that donut."

- Move! Get up from your desk every hour, do some squats, pull your belly in, and get 10,000 steps every day.

- Eat in a low glycemic fashion.

- Eat a wide variety of vegetables of multiple colors each day. They are low calorie and full of important nutrients. Include some fruit every day as well.

- Do resistance/weight work twice per week.

- Be on fructose patrol! Have the right size serving of fruit and be careful with dried fruit, which is full of fiber but also crystallized fructose.

- Your pleasure center is strong, but you are stronger, so you can beat it down by avoiding moderate to high glycemic carbs. After a week or two, it will be much easier.

- Try intermittent fasting, which is easier than you think, with this eating window: 11 a.m. to 8 p.m. or 10 a.m. to 7 p.m.

- Recruit your transverse abdominal muscle (TA). Pull that belly in!

- Eat and enjoy good fat.

- Eat healthy sources of protein like Goldilocks would do — not too much and not too little.

- Eat lots of fiber. You can get the fiber you need from eating a wide variety of vegetables in abundance, plus some fruit each day.

- Eat one tablespoon of ground flax seed per day.

- Prebiotic food is plant fiber, and the more, the better. Your microbiota will love you and that means you will feel better.

- Take 2,000 units of vitamin D-3.

- Do not use artificial sweeteners. They will only maintain your desire for sweets and damage your microbiota.

- Be purposeful in taking vitamins and supplements. Know what you are taking and why.

- Remember that a good diet outperforms a pill. Use a supplement as just that — a supplement to your diet.

- Ask your doctor if a baby aspirin is right for you. It is not for everyone.

- Dark chocolate? A healthy treat!

- Optimize your sleep! Get seven to eight hours per night.

- Avoid thriller TV or movies before bed. Play soothing music. Do not check your email!

- Sleep in a dark, quiet room. Turn off your smartphone and iPad and turn around the digital clock — they all give off a light that impacts your circadian rhythm.

- Power naps (about twenty minutes but not much more) can be good.

- Do not drink your calories, and instead, drink water when thirsty.

- Find time each day for stress relievers such as meditation or coherent breathing.

- Consider forgiveness. Your stress levels will go down.

- Take a few minutes before bed to consider at least one thing you are grateful for from the day. Consider keeping a notebook of these thoughts over time.

- HIIT is best but any exercise will help you maintain and enlarge your hippocampus and prefrontal cortex. It creates a reserve for when you may need it later.

- Minimize ingestion of alcohol. It is full of calories, affects your metabolism and sleep and rarely enhances your life

EPILOGUE

The poem below was given to Dr. Oken by a woman who had tried many times to work toward a healthy lifestyle. Each time she tried, she made a little progress and then she relapsed back to bad habits, but she kept trying until she found the way.

Autobiography in Five Short Chapters
By Portia Nelson

I walk down the street.

There is a deep hole in the sidewalk.

I fall in.

I am lost ... I am helpless.

It isn't my fault.

It takes forever to find a way out.

I walk down the same street.

There is a deep hole in the sidewalk.

I pretend I don't see it.

I fall in again.

I can't believe I am in the same place.

But it isn't my fault.

It still takes a long time to get out.

I walk down the same street.

There is a deep hole in the sidewalk.

I see it is there.

I still fall in … it's a habit.

My eyes are open.

I know where I am.

It is my fault.

I get out immediately.

I walk down the same street.

There is a deep hole in the sidewalk.

I walk around it.

I walk down another street.

Here are six things she told Dr. Oken that helped her attain good health:

1. Do what makes you happy. To the best of your ability, change, avoid or discard situations that cause you pain and unhappiness.

2. Visualize what you want to happen on a frequent basis.

3. Put positive pressure on yourself by sharing your ambitions with friends, family, and colleagues.

4. Use "inner talk" to remind yourself of what you want to accomplish.

5. You cannot always do it on your own, so enlist help.

6. Food diaries work!

We all have choices. The navigation of our lives is a journey, and we all share the same ultimate destination. The headwinds, tailwinds, and crosswinds are forever there, and we have to adjust our sails continuously to ensure the safest, healthiest and best ride. Getting there means changing bad habits to good ones, eating well, staying on the move, getting restorative rest, and finding peace and tranquility.

Jennifer made the choices she needed to make. It required Ellen's direct prodding, but Jennifer was convinced that the changes she made in her lifestyle had given her more energy, greater mental clarity, and a sense of wellness. It had started with "fear," — fear that she looked poorly and was losing her friends and her health — but after a few weeks on BOOM, she realized that she felt better, so much so that she no longer had any desire to revert back to her old ways. She felt like life was well worth living. She was frankly proud of herself. So were her friends, especially Ellen.

APPENDIX 1

Low Carb Meal Plan: 50 grams of total carbs

Day 1:
Late morning snack: 2-3 max hard-boiled eggs with serving of berries (½ cup)
Lunch: Salad using kale, spinach, or another dark leaf lettuce. Add lean protein: shrimp, chicken, pork, fish, or tofu
Other add-ons can include tomato, onion, broccoli, cucumber, asparagus, avocado, mushrooms, and bell pepper
Aged cheese - 1oz max (aim for aged cheese that is lower in lactose such as parmesan, gouda and swiss)
Nuts - ¼ cup max (pecans, brazil and macadamia are lowest in carbs)
*Try to make dressings at home to avoid extra ingredients hidden in store-bought dressings
Dinner: Baked, broiled or grilled lean protein of your choice, 2 servings (1 cup) of broccoli, asparagus or Brussels sprouts and a serving (½ cup) of squash or sweet potato (Make it sweet by tossing it with a little olive oil and sprinkle it with cinnamon.)

Day 2:
Late morning snack: 2-3 egg muffins (add in various vegetables/protein - zucchini, sundried tomato, kale, mushroom, spinach, red pepper, light cheese, turkey, or ham) plus a serving of berries (1/2 cup)
Lunch: Leftovers from dinner
Dinner: Stir fry (lean protein of choice) with vegetables (choose 1-2 servings of any green vegetable) and ⅓ cup of cauliflower rice
*Sauce recipe: Use 4 tbsp coconut aminos, tamari or soy sauce, 1 tsp fresh ginger, 2 tbsp coconut oil or olive oil and 1 tsp of garlic. Add red pepper flakes for an extra kick. Feel free to modify sauce to your personal taste. This is just a guideline.

Day 3:
Late morning snack: ½ apple with a serving of almond butter (no sugar added) or egg muffins plus a serving of fruit
Lunch: Leftovers from dinner
Dinner: Turkey and kale soup - feel free to modify the protein and vegetables

Day 4:
Late morning snack: Low-carb coconut cream pudding and a serving of berries
Lunch: Cup of canned wild tuna (or protein of choice) with a salad or leftovers from dinner
Dinner: Chicken (or protein of choice) skewers with rainbow cauliflower rice

Day 5:
Late morning snack: Overnight chia pudding with a serving of fruit
Lunch: Leftovers from dinner
Dinner: Frittata with fresh spinach - add in other vegetables and protein of choice, sprinkle with cheese and top with salsa

Day 6:
Late morning snack: Low-carb coconut cream pudding or low carb oatmeal with a serving of fruit
Lunch: Dark lettuce of choice salad with a serving of squash or sweet potato (½ cup), chopped cucumber, hard-boiled egg, ¼ avocado, serving of hemp seeds, ground pepper and a dressing from the list provided
Dinner: Roasted chicken with roasted veggies (Brussels sprouts, onions, carrots, radishes, broccoli, asparagus, fennel, onions)

Day 7:
Late morning snack: 2-3 egg muffins with a serving of berries or a kiwi
Lunch: Leftovers from dinner
Dinner: Spiralized zucchini (or another vegetable) noodles with tomato sauce and shrimp (or protein of choice) plus a side salad

Day 8:
Late morning snack: Breakfast stir fry or leftover egg muffins
Lunch: Leftovers or salad using kale, spinach, or another dark leaf lettuce. Add lean protein -shrimp, chicken, pork, fish, or tofu
Other add-ons can include tomato, onion, broccoli, cucumber, asparagus, avocado, mushrooms, and bell pepper
Aged cheese - 1 oz max (aim for aged cheese that is lower in lactose such as parmesan, gouda and swiss)
Nuts - ¼ cup max (pecans, brazil, macadamia-lowest in carbs)
*Try to make dressings at home to avoid extra ingredients hidden in store-bought dressings
Dinner: Salmon (or another type of fish) pockets plus a green vegetable (asparagus, broccoli, Brussels sprouts, sautéed spinach)

Day 9:
Late morning snack: Overnight chia pudding with a serving of fruit
Lunch: Leftovers from dinner or turkey roll-ups with cut-up vegetables
Dinner: Fish (or another lean protein) tacos with lettuce wraps and a green vegetable (asparagus, broccoli, Brussels sprouts, sautéed spinach, beans, cabbage, and cheese)
salsa or guacamole make a great topping

Day 10:
Late morning snack: Low-carb coconut cream or egg scramble
Lunch: Leftovers from dinner or canned wild tuna salad and a salad (can substitute for a side of cut of vegetables)
Dinner: Stir fry (protein of choice) with vegetables (choose 1-2 servings of any green vegetable and ⅓ cup of cauliflower rice)

Mid-Afternoon Snack Ideas: Combining a carbohydrate or vegetable with a protein makes a great balanced snack and keeps you full longer.

- Cut up celery, cucumber, broccoli, bell peppers and/or carrots with a serving of hummus, salsa, or guacamole
- Aged cheese - 1-2 oz
- Hard-boiled eggs
- Homemade kale chips – toss kale with a little olive oil and salt and bake at 325 degrees for a few minutes
- ½ cup of berries, a clementine, kiwi, ¼ cup of pomegranate seeds or ½ apple
- A handful of nuts - ¼ cup
- Homemade vanilla and cinnamon granola - low carb
- 1 oz of roasted turkey or ham (without added sugar) and celery
- Serving of nut butter (no added sugar)

Vegetarian Options: For any meal

- Swap out any animal protein with tofu, tempeh, or chickpeas
- Grilled portobello mushroom with vegetable and avocado
- Curried cauliflower chickpea bowl
- Tempeh stir fry with cashew nuts and vegetables
- Overnight chia seed pudding
- Low-carb oatmeal
- Fava bean and avocado salad

*For increase carb intake to 60 grams, clients may add an additional serving of fruit, hummus, nuts, or higher carb vegetable. Other options include a larger portion of starchy vegetables (i.e. butternut squash, carrots, bell peppers) during existing meals.

**Salad dressings make a great sauce for any of the dinners. It's a great way to add flavor!

APPENDIX 2

Exercise-High Intensity Interval Training (HIIT)

The exercise we use in the BOOM course is a type of HIIT that eventually transitions over time to a Tabata type of exercise. HIIT is an extension of work done by a Japanese exercise physiologist and Olympic speed skating coach Izumi Tabata, PhD. Tabata conducted numerous trials with his athletes, showing that HIIT improves aerobic and anaerobic performance in less time than traditional training,

In BOOM, we start with a warm-up on the spin bikes for about ten to fifteen minutes. In the early weeks, we then cycle as hard as we can with manageable resistance for thirty-second bursts, followed by an active recovery of ninety seconds. Initially, many participants find it challenging to complete all eight cycles. Nonetheless, we build both anaerobic and aerobic capacities rather quickly as we recruit ultra-fast white muscle fibers and create lactic acid byproducts, producing burning in our leg muscles, particularly the quadriceps and glute muscles.

Usually, by week three or four we progress towards a typical Tabata workout with accelerations followed by rest periods. Tabata's original work was a 2:1 ratio of work with rest. It can be effectively used in as little as four minutes with twenty seconds of hard work and ten seconds of rest! And we recommend doing this in addition to your weekly BOOM. A home workout suggestion is discussed on page 30.

In class, ultimately, we are striving for more cycles, up to fifteen, and less rest in active recovery. Depending on our class, by week twelve we may be doing twelve to fifteen of the thirty-second accelerations at a higher resistance, producing more output (watts) and sixty-second active recoveries. And so, in a relatively small amount of time, we are getting a sweaty, hard workout that boosts our metabolism for the rest of the day! You can do this yourself without our classes.

BOOM!

ACKNOWLEDGEMENTS

I began writing this book in 2012. But so often, life gets in the way of the best-made plans. In addition to my full-time practice, I was teaching clinical medicine at the University of Maryland, serving as the Medical Director of the Columbia Association, and conducting and publishing various medical studies. I also became distracted by a health problem — an unusual and difficult-to-diagnose illness that plagued one of my daughters. I turned to Steve Schimpff, my professor from medical school and training. In 1980, following my freshman year of medical school, I worked for Steve at the Baltimore Cancer Research Center, where he was the Head of Infectious Disease. Since that time, Steve has been a beacon of light in my life on many occasions, and this challenging period was no exception. With Steve's guidance, we got to the bottom of my daughter's illness, and thankfully, she made a complete recovery. Meanwhile, the unfinished draft of this book sat on my credenza for nearly six years.

I was elated when Steve agreed to help me finish writing this book. I am tremendously grateful for his friendship, guidance, and collaboration. I owe thanks to many friends and colleagues, too numerous to mention, who supported me in writing this book. Additionally, Sara Miller, the owner of Bare Nutrition, provided me with her 10-day meal plan in Appendix A; it is her creation and it works. I am also grateful to be part of the Persona Medical Advisory Board, as my associations with Persona has enriched my knowledge of nutrition; in my opinion, nutrition is the biggest single factor in attaining optimal health.

Finally, I am so grateful for the support of my family: my daughters — Rachel, Stacey, and Lindsey — along with my son-in-law, Steve, and my grandson, Jack. And of course, my best friend: my wife, Janet. She helps me to be a better person every day.

Harry A. Oken, MD, FACP

One day some 35 years ago, a University of Maryland first-year medical student named Harry Oken arrived at my office. He had a big smile and enthusiasm in his eyes. He said he would like to do a research project with me over the summer. I learned that he had a Master's Degree in microbiology; that suggested that he might be ideal to work on a serious issue we had in the cancer center at the time. We had a specialized sterile water system that was no longer producing sterile water. His project was to figure out what the problem was and then to figure out what we could do to solve it. He grabbed the project like a dog with a bone and shortly understood what this unusual organism was and to what it was resistant. Not long after, he figured out a solution — and it worked. Three years later, I encouraged him to submit this project for student research day. He was reluctant at first, having plenty of work to do as a senior medical student, but then he got into it. His project was judged the best of all. He was called out for the award at graduation.

He stayed at the University of Maryland for his internal medicine residency and then began a primary care practice in Columbia, Maryland. Over the years he's become recognized as one of the premier physicians in the community. We've stayed in contact and have had intermittent lunches together. One day he told me about a patient with an unusual Crohn's disease presentation that was not responding to standard therapy. By serendipity I had heard about a possible infectious cause, one discounted by gastroenterologists, just a month or so before. I told him about it and who he could contact for more information. Once again, he was like that dog with a bone — he immersed himself in the controversy and, along with curing his patient, he's become internationally recognized.

We both believe in the concept of "The Beginner's Mind." The beginner, not being an expert and therefore not knowing any better, is able to consider ideas that the specialist expert discounts because he or she already believes they know the answer. Two examples: Semmelweis was new at the obstetrics hospital but quickly realized that one of the two wards, the one with medical students, had a high death rate from "childbirth fever." Bacteria were not known then to cause disease, but he reasoned that the medical students should wash their hands after autopsies and before attending deliveries. The experts scoffed but the death rate plummeted. More recently, Drs. Barry Marshall and Robin Warren recognized that a bacterium named *Heliobacter pylori* caused most cases of peptic ulcer. For years, everyone scoffed, but ultimately, they were vindicated and won the Nobel Prize.

BOOM is a product of The Beginner's Mind. Dr. Oken put a program together that uses a scientific basis but that others had ignored. For example, he was well ahead of others in recognizing that a long overnight fast before high intensity interval exercise would have a profound metabolic impact. And it has worked. I've been exceedingly pleased to partner with him to develop this book.

Among those who deserve recognition:

Margaret Frazier has worked on the manuscript for each of my books, and she has done the same for this one, using her expert eye to edit our work and develop it for publication.

Hannah Reinsel, our graphic designer, developed the cover and the figures interspersed throughout the book. Her work makes the text much easier to read.

Carolyn Crist copyedited the manuscript, gave multiple important suggestions and completed the formatting.

Each week the Charlestown Writers Critique Group reviewed chapters and made important suggestions, including that it would be valuable to include an individual or two who had been through the program.

We are grateful to those notable individuals who have endorsed this book as well.

Most importantly, for my part, I want to thank Carol, my wife, for her advice. She listened as I described each chapter as they progressed and made critical recommendations. But more importantly, she has been the stable anchor for 56 years to whom I turn for support on a daily basis.

Stephen C. Schimpff, MD, MACP

AUTHOR BIOGRAPHIES

Harry A. Oken, MD, FACP, is a graduate of the University of Maryland with a B.S. in Zoology and an M.S. in Parasitology. In 1983, he graduated from the University of Maryland Medical School with Honors and is a member of Alpha Omega Alpha Honor Medical Society. He completed his internship and residency training at the University of Maryland, followed by an additional year as Chief Resident. He is board certified in the specialty of Internal Medicine by the American Board of Internal Medicine.

Dr. Oken continued to be involved in academic medicine and is an Adjunct Professor of Medicine at the University of Maryland. Every Wednesday afternoon for 28 years he ran the Ambulatory Internal Medicine Clinic for the Residency Program at the University of Maryland. He is a Fellow of the American College of Physicians.

Dr. Oken served for 14 years as Chairman of Medicine at Howard County General Hospital, where he is currently on staff as an Attending Physician. Dr. Oken has been listed in Best Doctors of America and has been a Baltimore's Top Doc as recently as 2018. His research interests are in a few areas, particularly nutrition and Crohn's disease, and has published in a variety of professional journals.

Dr. Oken's central theme with his patients is stressing good nutrition, attaining a healthy weight, getting regular exercise, and controlling stress. He continues to spearhead this theme as Medical Director for the Columbia Association. Dr. Oken has also been part of a health segment available for viewing at www.columbiamatters.org.

Stephen C. Schimpff, MD, MACP, is a graduate of Rutgers University and Yale School of Medicine with a career that spans over fifty years. He is a quasi-retired internist, researcher and professor of medicine at the University of Maryland School of Medicine and former professor in the School of Public Policy, founding director of the University of Maryland Greenebaum Cancer Center and former University of Maryland Medical Center chief executive officer. He is board certified in internal medicine, medical oncology and infectious diseases. He was recently elevated to Master, the highest honor bestowed by the American College of Physicians. His early career was at the National Cancer Institute and then the University of Maryland Medical School, where his research on preventing and treating infections in seriously ill cancer patients became acclaimed worldwide. He joined the University of Maryland Medical System as chief operating officer and later as chief executive officer of the flagship University of Maryland Medical Center. Since retirement, he has authored or co-authored six books for the general public on medical topics and co-authored a history of Canaan Valley, WV. He does a weekly TV show on health and wellness for the 2,000 residents of his retirement community. He and Carol, his wife of over 56 years, live in Maryland. Learn more about Dr. Schimpff's books, articles, and blog at www.megamedicaltrends.com.

EXCERPT FROM *LONGEVITY DECODED: THE 7 KEYS TO HEALTHY AGING*

Would you like to live a long time and be healthy until that last breath? It's possible. It's actually entirely up to you and all depends on your lifestyle. Modified appropriately, you can live a long and heathy life. Or you can predispose yourself to heart disease, cancer, diabetes, and Alzheimer's disease and have a shorter lifespan.

Lifespans have increased dramatically. For thousands of years, the average lifespan was no more than about 35 years. By the time of Abraham Lincoln, it had risen to about 45 years. Although many lived to their 80s and 90s and in good health, average lifespans were severely reduced by high rates of infant mortality, childhood illnesses, trauma and maternal deaths during deliveries. But by the late 1800's, lifespans began to rise rapidly. Perhaps most important was the advent of sanitary water and sewers systems, pasteurized milk, safe food handling practices and other public health measures. Add to these medical advances such as obstetrical care that reduced maternal mortality, reductions in infant mortality, vaccines to prevent childhood illnesses, trauma care to salvage young adults, antibiotics to treat infections, and improvements in medical care in general. This resulted in a major change in the top causes of death. In 1900 the three top three causes of death were infections – typhoid, tuberculosis and pneumonia. Today the top causes are chronic illnesses like heart disease, cancer, lung and diabetes. Importantly, each of these are largely ones that are the result of our lifestyle – how we live day-to-day. Today the average lifespan for men is about 76 years for women is about 81 years.

The aging process begins in our 20s and 30s with a loss of about 1 percent of each body organ and function each year. Too little to appreciate year to year, this inexorable process eventually results in brittle bones, weakened muscles, unsteady balance, disrupted cognition and slowed digestion, to name a few. As we age, the prevalence of these various chronic diseases rises rapidly. Sounds scary and suggests the elder years will be nothing but unpleasant.

The good news is that you can slow the aging process, prevent the diseases of aging and live a longer, healthier life. And if you get started early, the impact will compound over time just as saving dollars for retirement. To be clear, you will age and we all will die, but there is much you can do now.

There are seven key steps:

- Eat a healthy diet every day.
- Get adequate exercise.
- Manage chronic stress.
- Enhance your sleep.
- Don't smoke or over drink alcohol.
- Challenge your brain.
- Stay socially engaged.

Consider my great-great grandparents. They lived on a small farm and were largely self-sufficient. They ate two or three meals a day and never snacked. Food was locally sourced; vegetables and fruits were fresh and ripe; chickens spent the day in the fields. Fish came out of nearby streams and rivers, and meat came from animals hunted in the forests or grazed on the farm. There were no pesticides, no foods shipped thousands of miles, no meat from animals that were fattened with corn and soybeans, and no fish from fish farms. Candy, soda, and junk foods were almost unknown. There were no processed and packaged foods as we know them, and there were certainly no fast food restaurants — foods that are all heavily marketed today yet are inherently unhealthy but tasty with their ingredients of white flour, fat, sugar, and salt.

Everyone moved all day long, mostly outdoors; that was just natural. And much of that movement was hard work, the kind that kept muscles strong from lifting, bending, digging or hoeing. The kids were sent out, if not helping with farm chores, to play, and that play generally involved moving about.

Stress was present, of course, but somehow, they dealt with it and allowed it to "run off their backs." After a day of good food and plenty of movement, they slept easily and soundly from when the sun went down until the sun came up. Very few people smoked; cigarettes were not available. Alcohol was abundant, mostly homemade cider and beer and some wine.

Life was a constant challenge for the mind as well as the body. Families worked and played together and interacted with their neighbors. There were no radios, TVs or video games; families interacted with each other, and grandparents were honored and part of the family.

Many died early, as noted above, but many lived to a "ripe old age" yet rarely developed the chronic diseases of today — diabetes, lung cancer and heart disease.

Today Americans eat an average of 75 pounds of added sugar per year. Packaged in five-pound bags, that is 25 bags on your kitchen table — or 100 for a family of four. Of course, you don't eat that much added sugar but then someone else is consuming even more to make it average out. To top it off, we eat an inordinate amount of food made from white flour (e.g., cereal, cakes, pies, cookies, pastries, and pizza), which is digested directly to sugar. And of course, many of those foods are high in added sugar. Today we drive to work, stop for a pastry and latte, sit at a desk most of the day, eat a fast food lunch, enjoy an afternoon snack, drive home, call out for pizza, watch television and good to bed. Stress is everywhere – you need to check your emails and texts right up to bedtime. Your stress levels are off the charts. You probably don't smoke and that is good. You have all too little time for socializing with true friends. The alarm rings all too early and you are up and at it again.

What can you do? Will it really make a difference? Yes, focus on these seven key lifestyle modifications.

1 - Prepare meals from scratch; it actually does not take much time. Eat locally sourced, preferably organic vegetables and fruits in abundance. Vegetables should be the major components of your diet with a wide variety of types, colors, and textures to obtain all of the basic nutrients. Include dark leafy greens every day – spinach, collards, arugula, kale are good choices. Nuts, seeds, and foods such as avocados and olives have healthy oils, and omega-3 fatty acids are in wild caught fin fish such as salmon, mackerel and sardines. Avoid vegetable oils; use cold-pressed virgin olive oil instead. Choose chickens and eggs from hens that have been free ranged. Eat red meat sparingly and choose cuts from range fed animals that never saw a feed lot. And very importantly, avoid sugars like the plague and dramatically reduce your intake of foods made from white flour. It follows that you will cut back on processed foods and meals from fast food restaurants.

2 - Get up and move. Get 30 minutes of walking every day. That alone will have a huge impact on your immediate and long-term health. Add in a few sessions per week of strengthening ("resistance") exercises. Remember that "sitting is the new smoking." Park your car a distance from the building entrance. Take the stairs a few flights instead of the elevator. Get up from your computer and move around at least every half hour. Stand at your desk if possible. Spend less time sitting in a reclining chair watching TV at night.

3 - We all have chronic stress but many don't admit to it. Give some serious thought to your stresses. Eliminate the causes where possible and, for the remainder, consider ways to tamp it down. In addition to good food and regular exercise, along with adequate sleep, add in yoga, meditation, Tai Chi, coherent breathing or just a few moments

every so often to take a couple of deep breaths.

4 - To enhance sleep, don't snack after supper and for at least three hours before bedtime so your meal has been largely digested. Avoid reading or watching action or horror books, TV shows and movies before bedtime. Early in the evening, turn off your smartphone and don't look at texts, emails and Facebook. Instead, consider some soothing music before bed. Your bedroom needs to be pitch black with all your devices turned off. Keep to a schedule and remember that you need 7 ½ to eight hours of sleep each night. Don't listen to the friends who claim that they can get by on five or six hours; they are only fooling themselves.

5 - No tobacco. None, including vaping. And limit your alcohol consumption.

6 - Stimulate and challenge your brain. It needs to be used just like your muscles. Learn a new language or play an instrument. Do something creative like art or writing.

7 - Social engagement is important in slowing aging, preventing disease and enhancing a sense of wellness. Maintain connections with close friends.

Does this seem like a tall order? Perhaps, but just pick one or two areas to work at a time. Don't try to do it all at once. After a while you'll be doing great; you'll have more energy, more enthusiasm for life, much better health, and a longer, healthier lifespan. As an added bonus, if you get started early in adult life, you will reap the added benefits of compounding, just like saving for retirement. What could be better than that?

Learn more by reading *Longevity Decoded: The 7 Keys to Healthy Aging*, available on Amazon

1   Maffetone PB, Rivera-Dominguez I, and Laursen PB. Overfat adults and children in developed countries: the public health importance of identifying excess body fat. Frontiers in Public Health. 2017 Jul 24, http://bit.ly/2Z8AICj. Accessed August 10, 2019.

2   Ornish D. Quote form a video produced by Brian Vaszily ("Your Best Years Start Now") in which Ornish discusses some of the elements from *Undo It: How Simple Lifestyle Changes Can Reverse Most Chronic Diseases* written by Dean and Ann Ornish.

3   Patterson RE and Sears DD. Metabolic effects of intermittent fasting. Annu Rev Nutr. 2017 Aug 21;37:371-393. doi: 10.11467. http://bit.ly/2N3AF8F.

4   Sutton EF, et al. Early time-restricted feeding improves insulin sensitivity, blood pressure, and oxidative stress even without weight loss in men with prediabetes. Cell Metab. 2018 Jun 5;27(6):1212-1221.e3. doi: 10.1016/j.cmet.2018.04.010. http://bit.ly/33Ck6WZ.

5   Duncan F. The Ultimate Guide to Intermittent Fasting III – What Happens When You Fast? October 5, 2017. http://bit.ly/2MlUMzs. Accessed August 10, 2019.

6   Here is a video about the various types of fasting. https://amzn.to/2zAQFHD. Accessed August 10, 2019.

7   Di Francesco A, et al. Science. 2018 Nov 16;362(6416):770-775. doi: 10.1126/science.aau2095. https://tinyurl.com/y9ve8oen.

8   Germino D. Why Walking Will Make You More Productive and Creative – Philosophers, Writers, and Scientists Agree. Medium. Jan 31, 2019. http://bit.ly/306wHj6. Accessed August 10, 2019.

9   Kanaley J, et al. Human growth hormone response to repeated bouts of aerobic exercise, J Appl Physiol (1985). 1997

Nov;83(5):1756-61. http://bit.ly/2Z6HBs6.

[10] Owen N, et al. Sedentary behavior: emerging evidence for a new health risk. Mayo Clin Proc. 2010 Dec;85(12):1138-41. doi: 10.4065/mcp.2010.0444. http://bit.ly/2KPyWkr.

[11] Flegal K, et al. Association of all-cause mortality with overweight and obesity using standard body mass index categories - systematic review and meta-analysis, JAMA, 2013, 309: 71-82, doi:10.1001/jama.2012.113905. http://bit.ly/2KAUXVm.

[12] Obesity Responsible for More Deaths Than Smoking. The American Journal of Pharmacy Benefits. May 11, 2017. https://www.ajpb.com/news/obesity-responsible-for-more-deaths-than-smoking. Accessed August 10, 2019.

[13] Warren J, et al. A structured literature review on the role of mindfulness, mindful eating and intuitive eating in changing eating behaviours: effectiveness and associated potential mechanisms. Nutr Res Rev. 2017 Dec;30(2):272-283. doi: 10.1017/S0954422417000154. http://bit.ly/2OUcFHl

[14] Benson, H and Klipper, M. The Relaxation Response. New York: William Morrow, 1975, updated and expanded 2000. Print.

[15] Becker M, et al. Media multitasking is associated with symptoms of depression and social anxiety. Cyberpsychol Behav Soc Netw. 2013 Feb;16(2):132-5. doi: 10.1089/cyber.2012.0291. http://bit.ly/2OZCUMD.

[16] Also published in Schimpff, S. Longevity Decoded – The 7 Keys to Healthy Aging. Catonsville: Squire Publishing, 2018. Print.

[17] Rubin R. Whole-fat or nonfat dairy? The debate continues, JAMA. 2018 Dec 25;320(24):2514-2516. doi: 10.1001/jama.2018.17692. http://bit.ly/2H4IWp1.

[18] Shanahan F, et al. Feeding the microbiota: transducer of nutrient signals for the host. Gut. 2017;66(9):1709-1717. doi:1136/gutjnl-2017-313872

19   Haro C, et al. Two healthy diets modulate gut microbial community improving insulin sensitivity in a human obese population. J Clin Endocrinol Metab. 2016 Jan;101(1):233-42. doi: 10.1210/jc.2015-3351. 1210/jc.2015-3351.

20   Thaiss, C. Microbiome dynamics in obesity, Science. 2018;362: 903-904 http://bit.ly/2z1yn1p.

21   Thaiss C, et al, Hyperglycemia drives intestinal barrier dysfunction and risk for enteric infection. *Science.* 2018;359: 1376-1383.doi 10.1126/science.aar3318. http://bit.ly/306z1qk.

22   Fu J, et al. The gut microbiome contributes to a substantial proportion of the variation in blood lipids. Circ Res. 2015 Oct 9;117(9):817-24. doi: 10.1161/CIRCRESAHA.115.306807. 1161/CIRCRESAHA.115.306807

23   Pedersen HK, et al. Human gut microbes impact host serum metabolome and insulin sensitivity. Nature. 2016 Jul 21;535(7612):376-81. 10.1038/nature18646

24   Menni C, et al. Gut microbial diversity is associated with lower arterial stiffness in women. Eur Heart J. 2018 Jul 1;39(25):2390-2397. doi: 10.1093/eurheartj/ehy226. 1093/eurheartj/ehy226

25   Rajindrajit S, et al. Childhood constipation as an emerging public health problem. World J Gastroenterol. 2016 Aug 14;22(30):6864-75. doi: 10.3748/wjg.v22.i30.6864. 10.3748/wjg.v22.i30.6864

26   Arterburn LM, et al. Distribution, interconversion, and dose response of n-3 fatty acids in humans. Am J Clin Nutr. 2006 Jun;83(6 Suppl):1467S-1476S. doi: 10.1093/ajcn/83.6.1467S. http://bit.ly/2TD3WYO.

27   Greger M. Flax Seeds and Breast Cancer Prevention. April 5, 2013, volume 12. Video. http://bit.ly/2KN2wXT. Accessed August 10, 2019.

28   Greger M. Flax Seeds Versus Prostate Cancer. March 25, 2013, volume 12. Video. http://bit.ly/2Ha9AwB. Accessed August 10, 2019.

29   Armitage H. Diabetic-level glucose spikes seen in healthy people, Stanford Medicine News Center, July 24, 2018. https://stan.md/2KCpJgB. Accessed August 10, 2019.

30   Dunster G, et al. Sleep more in Seattle: later school start times are associated with more sleep and better performance in high school students. Sci Adv. 2018 Dec 12;4(12):eaau6200. doi: 10.1126/sciadv.aau6200. http://bit.ly/2YTw5ko.

31   The Nutrition Source, Harvard School of Public Health, Shining the Spotlight on Trans Fats, http://bit.ly/2P1Pw62. Accessed August 10, 2019.

32   U.S. Senate Select Committee on Nutrition and Human Needs, Dietary Goals for the United States, US Government Printing office, 1977. http://bit.ly/30bL0Tr. Accessed August 10, 2019.

33   Mozaffarian D and Ludwig, S. Dietary guidelines in the 21st century – a time for food. JAMA. 2010 Aug 11;304(6):681-2. doi: 10.1001/jama.2010.1116. http://bit.ly/2N6KgeF.

34   Public Health Service, US Dept of Health and Human Services, Healthy People 2000, National Health Promotion and Disease Prevention Objective, 1991. http://bit.ly/2KQCpiJ.

35   Pett KD, et al. Ancel Keys and the Seven Countries Study: An Evidence-based Response to Revisionist Histories. Commissioned by The True Health Initiative. August, 2017. http://bit.ly/31NX4Ln.

36   Michaëlsson K. Milk intake and risk of mortality and fractures in women and men: cohort studies. BMJ. 2014 Oct 28;349:g6015. doi: 10.1136/bmj.g6015. http://bit.ly/33FLRyc.

37   Suez J, et al. Artificial sweeteners induce glucose intolerance by altering the gut microbiota. Nature. 2014 Oct 9;514(7521):181-6. doi: 10.1038/nature13793. https://go.nature.com/33E5qXy.

38   Nettleton J, et al, Diet soda intake and risk of incident metabolic syndrome and type 2 diabetes in the multi-ethnic study of atherosclerosis. Diabetes Care. 2009 Apr;32(4):688-94. doi: 10.2337/dc08-1799. 10.2337/dc08-1799

39   Sesso HD, et al. Multivitamins in the prevention of

cardiovascular disease in men: the Physicians Health Study II randomized controlled trial. JAMA 2012;308:1751–60. https://bit.ly/2MGS5WQ

40 Rowan, J. Is Sunscreen the New Margarine? Outside. January 10, 2019. http://bit.ly/2TJ7ysA. Accessed August 10, 2019.

41 McGreevey S and Morrison, M, Study confirms vitamin D protects against colds and flu, The Harvard Gazette, Feb 15, 2017. http://bit.ly/33D6MBI. Accessed August 10, 2019.

42 Rosen C. Vitamin D insufficiency. N Engl J Med. 2011; 364:248-254. DOI: 10.1056/NEJMcp1009570. http://bit.ly/2P0QXBB.

43 Heaney R. Vitamin D – baseline status and effective dose. N Engl J Med. 2012; 367:77-78. DOI: 10.1056/NEJMe1206858. http://bit.ly/30dQCN9.

44 Hewlings SJ and Kalman DS. Curcumin: review of its effects on human health. Foods. 2017 Oct 22;6(10). pii: E92. doi: 10.3390/foods6100092. 10.3390/foods6100092.

45 Shoba G, et al. Influence of piperine on the pharmacokinetics of curcumin in animals and human volunteers. Planta Med. 1998 May;64(4):353-6. http://bit.ly/2N7yCjX.

46 Manson J, et al. Marine n-3 fatty acids and prevention of cardiovascular disease and cancer. N Engl J Med. 2019; 380:23-32. DOI: 10.1056/NEJMoa1811403. http://bit.ly/2YXgTTy

47 Bhatt D, et al. Cardiovascular risk reduction with icosapent ethyl for hypertriglyceridemia. N Engl J Med. N Engl J Med. 2019 Apr 25;380(17):1678. doi: 10.1056/NEJMc1902165. http://bit.ly/2TEbCKB

48 Watson, J, Reviewed by: Anya Romanowski, MS, RD. Vitamin K2 Steps Into the Spotlight for Bone and Heart Health. Medscape. October 10, 2018. https://tinyurl.com/y2qun233. Accessed August 10, 2019.

49 Greger M. Are Calcium Supplements Safe? November 16, 2015, volume 27. Video. http://bit.ly/2Z5fYLW. Accessed August 10, 2019.

50   Zheng S and Roddick A. Association of aspirin use for primary prevention with cardiovascular events and bleeding events – a systematic review an meta-analysis. JAMA. 2019; 321: 277-287 doi: 10.1001/jama.2018.20578. http://bit.ly/2z1dtzy.

51   Gaziano J. Aspirin for primary prevention – clinical considerations in 2019. JAMA. 2019 Jan 22;321(3):253-255. doi: 10.1001/jama.2018.20577. http://bit.ly/33Czjrh.

52   McNeil JJ, et al. Effect of aspirin on all-cause mortality in the healthy elderly. N Engl J Med. 2018; 379:1519-1528. DOI: 10.1056/NEJMoa1803955. http://bit.ly/308vV59.

53   Collins F. An aspirin a day for older people doesn't prolong healthy lifespan. NIH Directors Blog, Sept 25, 2018. http://bit.ly/33D9cjR

54   Rothwell PM, et al. Effects of aspirin on risks of vascular events and cancer according to bodyweight and dose: analysis of individual patient data from randomised trials. Lancet. 2018 Aug 4;392(10145):387-399. doi: 10.1016/S0140-6736(18)31133-4. http://bit.ly/2OVfQ1F.

55   Jackson S, et al. Is there a relationship between chocolate consumption and symptoms of depression? A cross-sectional survey of 13,626 US adults. Depression and Anxiety, 2019; DOI: 10.1002/da.22950. https://bit.ly/2MFapzx. Accessed October 14, 2019.

56   Greger M. Can hydration affect our mood? Nutritionfacts.org, September 12 2017, http://bit.ly/31JTXE1. Accessed August 10, 2019.

57   Xi B, et al. Relationship of alcohol consumption to all-cause, cardiovascular, and cancer-related mortality in U.S. adults. J Am Coll Cardiol. 2017 Aug 22;70(8):913-922. doi: 10.1016/j.jacc.2017.06.054. http://bit.ly/2Z6XeLS.

58   Environmental Working Group, 2018 Shopper's Guide to Pesticides in Produce. http://bit.ly/2Mlrf8L. Accessed August 10, 2019.

Made in the USA
Middletown, DE
30 May 2023

31220146R00135